Exposure to Psychotropic Medications and Other Substances during Pregnancy and Lactation

A HANDBOOK FOR HEALTH CARE PROVIDERS

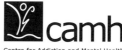

camh
Centre for Addiction and Mental Health
Centre de toxicomanie et de santé mentale
A Pan American Health Organization/
World Health Organization Collaborating Centre

MOTHERISK
Treating the Mother –
Protecting the Unborn

Library and Archives Canada Cataloguing in Publication

Exposure to psychotropic medications and other substances during pregnancy and lactation: a handbook for health care providers/Centre for Addiction and Mental Health (CAMH).

Includes bibliographical references and index.
ISBN: 978-0-88868-601-5 (print)   978-0-88868-599-5 (PDF)   978-0-88868-600-8 (HTML)

1. Psychotropic drugs. 2. Fetus—Effect of drugs on. 3. Perinatal pharmacology. 4. Developmental toxicology. 5. Pregnant women—Drug use. 6. Mothers—Drug use. I. Centre for Addiction and Mental Health

RG627.6.D79E96 2007   618.3'2   C2007-903683-X

Printed in Canada

For information on other CAMH publications or to place an order, please contact:

Sales and Distribution
Tel.: 1 800 661-1111 or 416 595-6059 in Toronto
E-mail: publications@camh.net

Website: www.camh.net

The following people produced this handbook:
Project lead: Betty Dondertman, CAMH
Development: Susan Rosenstein, CAMH; Elizabeth Scott
Editorial: Martha Ayim, CAMH; Nick Gamble, CAMH
Design: Nancy Leung, CAMH
Typesetting: Philip Sung Design Associates
Print production: Christine Harris, CAMH; Annie McFarlane, CAMH; Lawrie Korec
Webinar developer: Rosalicia Rondon, CAMH

P134/3410/11-07

Acknowledgments

Production of this handbook has been made possible through a financial contribution from Health Canada. The views expressed herein do not necessarily represent the views of Health Canada.

The partners

The **Centre for Addiction and Mental Health (CAMH)** in Ontario is the largest addiction and mental health organization in North America, combining clinical care services, health promotion, education and research. CAMH produces resources—including online and classroom courses, workshops, seminars and publications—for front-line workers in addiction and mental health, for primary care providers, for helping professionals and for the general public. For more information about CAMH, visit www.camh.net.

The **Motherisk Program** at the Hospital for Sick Children in Toronto is a clinical, research and teaching program dedicated to antenatal drug, chemical and disease risk counselling. Created in 1985, Motherisk provides evidence-based information and guidance about the safety or risk to the developing fetus or infant of maternal exposure to drugs, chemicals, diseases, radiation and environmental agents. For more information about Motherisk, visit www.motherisk.org.

The contributors

Adrienne Einarson, RN, is an experienced nursing professional, with specialties in midwifery and psychiatry. An active member of Motherisk's research team, Ms. Einarson's main research interests are psychiatry, nausea and vomiting of pregnancy, and alternative medicine. She also conducts studies that examine the perception of risk and decision-making determinants regarding the use of drugs during pregnancy. She has published numerous papers in peer-reviewed journals in these areas, many on the safety of psychotropic drug use in pregnancy.

Meldon Kahan, MD, CCFP, FRCPC, is an associate professor and researcher in the Department of Family Medicine at the University of Toronto. He is also medical director of the Addiction Medicine Service at St. Joseph's Health Centre in Toronto, and an author and editor of two textbooks on addiction. Dr. Kahan is also a staff physician at CAMH.

Alice Ordean, MD, CCFP, MHSC, is medical director of the Toronto Centre for Substance Use in Pregnancy (T-CUP) and one of the few physicians in Ontario with expertise in both addiction and primary care obstetrics. She is also the physician representative on Pregnets, a prenatal smoking cessation project. Dr. Ordean has presented on many occasions to care providers at various hospitals and organizations, including the departments of obstetrics and gynecology at Mount Sinai Hospital in Toronto, Toronto East General Hospital and Trillium Health Centre, as well as the Toronto Children's Aid Society and Toronto Public Health.

Kate Tschakovsky, MSW, RSW, has worked in a variety of community settings, including women's shelters, programs for young offenders and prisons. At CAMH, she has been involved in a range of areas, including methadone treatment, women's and youth programming and HIV services; she currently works in the Schizophrenia Program. Ms. Tschakovsky has written for and collaborated extensively on several treatment-related manuals and books. Her current interests are the evaluation and implementation of harm reduction strategies in addiction services, and concurrent disorders.

Wende Wood, RPH, BA, BSP, BCPP, is a psychiatric pharmacist registered through the Board of Pharmaceutical Specialties in the United States. She is the first person in Ontario and the 10th in Canada to achieve this designation. Ms. Wood is the Drug Information and Drug Use Evaluation Pharmacist at CAMH. She is widely published and frequently gives lectures and interviews across North America on psychiatric medications and substance use issues.

The reviewers

Special thanks to the following professionals who reviewed early versions or sections of this handbook and provided valuable insight and feedback: **Heather Bennett**, BPHARM, PHD, Ontario; **Yousef Botros**, BSCPHM, Ontario; **Ariel Dalfen**, MD, FRCPC, Ontario; **Alicja Fishell**, BSC, MD, FRCPC, Ontario; **Jennifer Fitzpatrick**, British Columbia; **Gabriella Herr**, BSCN, RN(EC), PHCNP, MN, Ontario; **Ryan Huffman**, BA, Ontario; **Tanya Kotowycz**, BSCPHM, Ontario; **Ginny Lane**, RD, Saskatchewan; **Marielle Layton**, MLIS, Alberta; **Melody Mann**, BA, BSW, Ontario; **Kimberly McDougall**, BSCPHM, Alberta; **Royanne Mitchell**, RN, Ontario; **Sridhar Nilam**, MBBS, CCFP, CASAM, Ontario; **Vinay Phokeo**, BSCPHM, MSC, Ontario; **Nancy Poole**, MA, PHD candidate, British Columbia; **Brenda Stankiewicz**, BSCN, PHN, Ontario; **Lucy Van Wyk**, MSW, RSW, Ontario; **Adil Virani**, BSCPHM, PHARMD, FCSHP, British Columbia; **Nese Yuksel**, BSCPHM, PHARMD, Alberta.

We also thank members of the PRIMA National Committee: **Ron Abrahams**, MD, FCFP, British Columbia; **Lisa Graves**, MD, CCFP, Quebec; **Georgia Hunt**, MD, British Columbia; **Meldon Kahan**, MD, CCFP, FRCPC, Ontario; **Lisa Lefebvre**, MDCM, CCFP, Ontario; **Margaret Leslie**, DIPCS, CPSYCHASSOC, Ontario; **Nick Leyland**, BSC, MD, FRCSC, FSOGC, Ontario; **Deana Midmer**, BSCN, MED, EDD, Ontario; **Patricia Mousmanis**, MD, CCFP, FCFP, Ontario; **Alice Ordean**, MD, CCFP, MHSC, Ontario; **Sarah Payne**, RN, MA, British Columbia; **Melanie Smith**, MA, Ontario.

Contents

Preface

We know that 25 per cent of Canadians smoke,[1] five per cent drink alcohol daily and 10 per cent report symptoms consistent with alcohol or illegal drug dependence. We can conclude, then, that many of the over 400,000 Canadian women who give birth each year may have used such substances before they knew they were pregnant.

In addition, approximately 10 to 15 per cent of women between the ages of 25 and 44 experience depression. One study[2] found that 6.6 per cent of pregnant women between the ages of 15 and 45 had been on an antidepressant during the year prior to conception. Given these figures, a substantial number of these women are likely to be taking antidepressants when they become pregnant. When women who are taking a psychotropic medication find out they are pregnant, they may assume they need to stop treatment. However, while some psychotropics do have effects on the baby, the negative effects of untreated illness can often—as in the case of depression—be very serious.

The health care provider's challenge is to know the true risks and benefits, to both the mother and her fetus or baby, of taking versus stopping the use of a medication or other substance. Yet the average health care provider is not well equipped to give the best advice to women who are pregnant or breastfeeding and exposed to psychotropics.

- "Is it ever safe to drink alcohol when breastfeeding?"
- "What are the risks to the baby if the mother uses cannabis while pregnant or breastfeeding?"
- "Are the effects of smoking different during pregnancy versus during breastfeeding?"
- "What is the effect of cocaine on the fetus or neonate?"
- "If a woman stops taking an antidepressant when she becomes pregnant, what will be the effect on her and the fetus?"
- "Can a woman safely breastfeed her baby when taking codeine?"

The information in this handbook will provide practitioners with evidence-based facts and recommendations on these and many other questions.

In 2003, CAMH and Motherisk collaborated on *Is It Safe for My Baby? Risks and Recommendations for the Use of Medication, Alcohol, Tobacco and Other Drugs during Pregnancy and Breastfeeding*, which was written for women and the general public. We know that health care providers will also benefit from a convenient source of evidence-based information on this topic.

Our goal with this publication is to help primary care physicians, psychiatrists, pharmacists, obstetricians, midwives, public health nurses and nurse practitioners provide the best advice, information and care to women who are taking psychotropic medications or other substances during pregnancy and postpartum. Medications and other substances discussed in this handbook have been chosen because of their psychotropic qualities: they all affect brain chemistry and functioning. Drugs and substances that are not psychotropic, that are not used during pregnancy, or about whose effects there is not enough documented evidence (e.g., herbal remedies) are not included.

The sections on psychotropic medications and other substances are organized alphabetically by drug or drug category. When talking about specific drugs, we have included the generic and brand names. The examples given are some of the most commonly used drugs, but do not necessarily include all drugs in that category. An index of drugs beginning on page 107 lists all the drug categories and generic and brand names used in this handbook.

The information in this handbook is based on the most recent research, and is current as of October 2007.

We trust you will find this handbook useful.

On behalf of CAMH and Motherisk
Betty Dondertman, project lead, CAMH
October 2007

References

1. Statistics Canada. (2003, June). . . . *Au Courant*. Ottawa: Minister of Industry. (Catalogue No. 82-005-XIE). Available: www.statcan.ca/english/freepub/82-005-XIE/82-005-XIE2002003.pdf. Accessed June 25, 2007.
2. Ramos, É., Oraichi, D., Rey, É., Blais, L. & Bérard, A. (2007). Prevalence and predictors of antidepressant use in a cohort of pregnant women. *British Journal of Obstetrics and Gynaecology*. Published OnlineEarly June 12, 2007. Available: www.blackwell-synergy.com/doi/abs/10.1111/j.1471-0528.2007.01387.x. Accessed June 25, 2007.

General Issues and Background

Myths and facts

A lot of misinformation exists concerning drug use during pregnancy and breastfeeding. Much of this information is passed on to the general public through the media, well-meaning family and friends, and even health care practitioners. Why does this misleading information exist? Prior to the 1950s, it was thought that a pregnant woman developed a "placental barrier" through which nothing that would hurt the fetus could pass. As a result, during that era, there was little concern over what a woman may be exposed to during pregnancy. Then the thalidomide tragedy occurred and the common belief, as often happens, swung to the other extreme. Today, it is widely believed that most substances can harm the fetus or baby, and that women should not be exposed to any medication or other substance while pregnant or breastfeeding. Common sense should tell us, however, that the truth lies somewhere in between.

Here are some common myths about exposure during pregnancy and breastfeeding, and some facts to dispel those myths.

Depression and other mental illnesses during pregnancy

Myth: Pregnancy has a protective effect against mental illness. While pregnant, a woman is shielded from depression and another mental illnesses.

Fact: Pregnancy has no protective effect whatsoever. Some women who already have a mental illness are at a higher risk for relapse if they stop taking their medication.

Medication use in general during pregnancy and breastfeeding

Myth: It's important to always use the medication that has the most safety data available.

Fact: While this sounds like good information, if the drug with the most safety data is not effective for a particular woman or if she is taking a different drug when she becomes pregnant, this would not be the best advice.

Myth: It is dangerous to take medications while breastfeeding.

Fact: Many drugs can be taken while breastfeeding without harm to the infant. The American Academy of Pediatrics considers excretion of less than 10 per cent of a drug into the breast milk to be compatible with breastfeeding.

Antidepressant, antipsychotic and benzodiazepine use during pregnancy

Myth: These drugs should be used during pregnancy only in the most severe cases.

Fact: In general, if a woman is being treated successfully with pharmacotherapy for mental illness before she becomes pregnant, her treatment should continue throughout pregnancy as well. Untreated depression and other mental illnesses—regardless of the severity—can harm both the mother and her fetus or baby.

Antiepileptic and lithium use during pregnancy

Myth: Since these drugs have been found to cause birth defects, they should be avoided during pregnancy.

Fact: Because these drugs are used to treat serious illnesses (e.g., epilepsy and bipolar disorder), the benefits and risks associated with their use, and with cessation of their use, must always be weighed before making any changes. For example, the risk that a baby will have a birth defect is minimal; often the risk of the mother relapsing or experiencing untreated illness is more serious.

Alcohol use during pregnancy and breastfeeding

Myth: A woman who has had a few drinks prior to finding out that she is pregnant will have a baby with fetal alcohol spectrum disorder.

Fact: There is no evidence to support this claim. In the "all-or-nothing period"—between six and 12 days after fertilization but before implantation (i.e., before the woman knows she is pregnant)—either injuries to the conceptus (whether or not they were caused by exposure to alcohol) will result in the woman having a spontaneous abortion, or the woman will continue to have a normal, healthy pregnancy.

Myth: If a woman who has been drinking during her pregnancy decides to stop drinking, it will be too late to prevent damage to her baby.

Fact: It's never too late for a pregnant woman to stop drinking because the less alcohol she consumes, the lower the risk of adverse effects on her baby.

Myth: A woman should never take a drink when she is breastfeeding her baby.

Fact: If a woman plans to have a few drinks, she can minimize the amount of alcohol secreted into her breast milk by estimating how long it will take until the alcohol is excreted from her body. (See Figure 4 on page 42 for an algorithm designed specifically for making this calculation.)

Smoking during pregnancy

Myth: To prevent any harmful effects that could put the fetus or child at risk, a woman must completely quit smoking during pregnancy.

Fact: Smoking is extremely addictive and some women find it tremendously difficult to quit. However, by reducing the number of cigarettes smoked each day, adverse effects can be minimized. Therefore, women should be encouraged and supported to cut down on the quantity smoked.

Myth: A woman who smokes in her third trimester will lower the birth weight of her baby and will therefore have an easier labour.

Fact: While smoking in the third trimester may lower a baby's birth weight to some extent, the amount is probably not enough to significantly ease labour. Further, low birth weight can result in potentially significant complications for the baby.

Cocaine use versus alcohol or tobacco use during pregnancy

Myth: "Crack babies" grow into severely damaged children whose needs drain the health care and social service systems.

Fact: While exposure to cocaine may affect the fetus, studies suggest that neonates exposed to cocaine in utero may experience less severe effects than neonates born to mothers who used alcohol regularly or excessively, or who smoked half a pack of cigarettes a day during pregnancy. In fact, alcohol consumption during pregnancy is the leading preventable cause of neurodevelopmental deficits in Canada.

Opioid use during pregnancy

Myth: Opioids shouldn't be used in pregnancy. If a woman finds out she's pregnant, she should stop using opioids immediately.

Fact: A woman shouldn't necessarily stop taking opioids when she discovers she is pregnant. In fact, withdrawal effects from opioid cessation can trigger uterine contractions that, in the first trimester, can lead to spontaneous abortion (or, in the third trimester, can lead to premature labour).

Key principles

Several principles can be integrated into clinical approaches to working with pregnant or breastfeeding women who use psychotropic medications or other substances. These principles will not necessarily apply equally to all women. Some women taking psychotropic medication may live in a stable environment that includes a support network, safe housing and secure employment. Some women may have substance use problems and endure violence and poverty. Some women may live with both substance use and mental health problems. Awareness of the key principles will allow providers to apply the most relevant principles to individual women in their care.

Consider the determinants of health

When assessing a woman's health before, during and after pregnancy, practitioners need a holistic approach that—in addition to substance use and mental health problems—takes into consideration the determinants of health. These determinants include:[1,2]

- access to health care
- income and socio-economic status
- social inclusion and exclusion
- social support networks
- early childhood care
- education and literacy
- working conditions
- employment and job security
- housing
- food security and nutrition
- physical environments (e.g., safe water, clean air, adequate transportation systems)
- personal health practices and coping skills
- biology and genetic endowment
- gender
- culture.

Women whose care takes into account their overall home environment, social support systems and other factors that affect their day-to-day living benefit more than those whose drug use alone is taken into account. For example, many women at risk of using substances during pregnancy face numerous social and economic stresses. Unemployment, violence, poverty and other issues may not only blur the importance of stopping substance use and seeking health care services, but may even create an environment where substance use serves as a benefit by numbing them to some of the realities of their lives. It is unreasonable to request that a woman stop using substances without addressing the multiple stressors that challenge a woman's successful cessation.[3]

Provide women-centred care

Interventions with pregnant and breastfeeding women who use substances have traditionally focused on fetal health; women-centred care is an approach to clinical encounters that places value on a woman's needs in the context of her life circumstances, such as whether she is experiencing violence or whether the pregnancy was wanted.[3,4] This requires a holistic approach to health, including mental and physical health, as well as an awareness of the socio-economic context of a woman's life. A women-centred approach focuses on a woman's long-term health and intrinsic reasons for change—in this way it addresses longer-term motivation (i.e., beyond pregnancy and breastfeeding) for becoming and remaining abstinent from substances. Understanding how a woman's unique situation impacts her substance use and mental health will allow practitioners to offer interventions tailored to individual women's realities, priorities and needs. The British Columbia Centre of Excellence for Women's Health proposes a women-centred model that encompasses a wide range of considerations (see Figure 1).

Fight stigma

The prejudice and discrimination at the heart of stigma affect the extent to which pregnant women with substance use and/or mental health problems receive both prenatal and postnatal care. A woman who is

Figure 1: Providing women-centred care

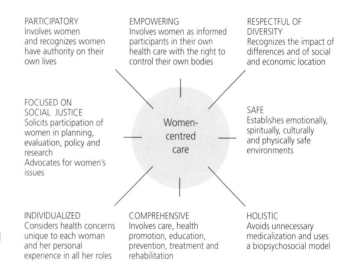

PARTICIPATORY
Involves women and recognizes women have authority on their own lives

EMPOWERING
Involves women as informed participants in their own health care with the right to control their own bodies

RESPECTFUL OF DIVERSITY
Recognizes the impact of differences and of social and economic location

FOCUSED ON SOCIAL JUSTICE
Solicits participation of women in planning, evaluation, policy and research
Advocates for women's issues

Women-centred care

SAFE
Establishes emotionally, spiritually, culturally and physically safe environments

INDIVIDUALIZED
Considers health concerns unique to each woman and her personal experience in all her roles

COMPREHENSIVE
Involves care, health promotion, education, prevention, treatment and rehabilitation

HOLISTIC
Avoids unnecessary medicalization and uses a biopsychosocial model

Reprinted with permission from Poole, N. & Greaves, L. (Eds.) (2007). *Highs & Lows: Canadian Perspectives on Women and Substance Use.* Toronto: Centre for Addiction and Mental Health. Copyright © 2001 British Columbia Centre of Excellence for Women's Health.

thought to be endangering the health of her fetus or baby (e.g., by not abstaining from substances or not following a doctor's or midwife's advice) has typically been considered a "bad" mother. This stigma can contribute to women with substance use and mental health problems keeping their symptoms and problems secret. As a result, they may avoid getting the help they need.

Statistics Canada reports that only 32 per cent of people with a mental health problem seek professional help;[5] this means the majority receive no care at all. A pregnant woman who uses substances has the additional fear that disclosing information may lead to losing her child to child protection services (e.g., Children's Aid Society or Children's Services). As a result, she may minimize important issues that are fundamental to developing an effective treatment plan with her doctor.

In addition to compromized medical care, stigma can affect other areas of a woman's life, including limiting her ability to secure employment; find safe and stable housing; be accepted by her family, friends and community; make friends or have other long-term relationships; and take part in social activities.

People with substance use and mental health problems often internalize prejudice and discrimination. This self-stigma leads them to believe the external messages from others and the media. The guilt and shame that often result from stigma can lead to low self-esteem, social isolation, weaker support networks, increased poverty, depression, loss of hope for recovery, and even suicide. These outcomes can clearly affect a woman's ability to cope with her own and her child's care, both during pregnancy and afterward.

To help mitigate stigma's effects as much as possible, providers can:

- be aware of attitudes and behaviour. Prejudice and discrimination are passed on by society and reinforced by family, friends and the media. Challenging one's own and others' thinking can help to ensure that people are seen as unique human beings, not as labels or stereotypes.

- be mindful about language. The way a person speaks can affect the way others think and speak. It is important to use accurate and sensitive words when talking to and about people with substance use and mental health problems. For example, using the phrase "a person with an addiction" instead of "a drug user" puts the person first and then identifies the issue she may have, rather than dehumanizing a person and defining her by the substance use.

- provide outreach. Since many women with substance use and mental health problems are stigmatized and marginalized (e.g., by social exclusion, low socio-economic status, lack of formal education), it is important to ensure that women who do not present to health care providers are also reached. (See "An Example of Key Principles in Action" on pages 8 to 10 for an inspiring illustration of an outreach program.)

Examine partner/social support

Few interventions focus on a woman's partner or social environment, yet both cessation and relapse are affected by the presence of people who use substances in close proximity to the woman,[3] as well as the amount of support a woman has. It is important to acknowledge the presence of others who use substances in a woman's life and to determine the dynamics of those relationships. When exploring a partner's behaviour, it is crucial to acknowledge potential power, control and abuse issues in a way that ensures the woman's safety. Validate a woman's entitlement to social support—because of stigma and the resulting shame, a woman may not feel that she deserves help. Encourage women to find appropriate support (e.g., confiding in a trusted friend, seeking a referral for additional services).

Integrate a harm reduction philosophy

Harm reduction—any program or policy that aims to reduce the harmful consequences of substance use without requiring the cessation, or even necessarily the reduction, of drug use—offers a practical approach to managing addiction.[6] These strategies prioritize the goals of a person who uses substances, with an emphasis on immediate and realizable goals. Harm reduction initiatives are flexible, recognizing individual differences and the potential for a woman to re-evaluate her goals. They provide a maximum range of treatment options such as drug substitution, drug maintenance and interventions that adopt safer methods of use. A woman's decision to use drugs is acknowledged as a personal choice, for which she takes responsibility. In this way, harm reduction strategies can help circumvent the stigma associated with substance use because they take a non-judgmental approach to people who use drugs.

Harm reduction can also mean helping women reduce or prevent the harm associated with other high-risk behaviours (e.g., unsafe sex) or environments (e.g., physical abuse, unsafe housing).[3] By examining behaviours and environments, and offering information, providers encourage women to make healthier and safer choices for themselves, even if complete abstinence is not feasible, and support them in finding safer environments. Effective therapeutic intervention includes recognizing that some women may currently be ambivalent about their substance use or resistant to abstinence.

Examples of harm reduction choices include:

- safer injection use and methadone maintenance treatment
- nutritional improvements, which may moderate the effects of substance use
- other health-enhancing practices, such as safer sex, more physical activity and using stress reduction techniques.

Identify concurrent disorders

Recent research[7-11] has indicated a high prevalence of concurrent disorders—co-occurring substance-related and mental disorders. It is estimated that in Canada, between 40 and 60 per cent of people with severe mental illness will develop a substance use disorder in their lifetime.[11] And opioid dependence is associated with almost every major mental illness (most commonly with mood and anxiety disorders, eating disorders and personality disorders). If concurrent disorders are not recognized and treated, negative effects can include:

- the risk of harmful interactions between psychotropic medications and other substances
- misinterpretation of symptoms (e.g., what seems to be a sign of substance use or withdrawal may actually indicate a mental health problem)
- a woman dropping out of treatment prematurely, thereby increasing the risk of harm to herself and her fetus or infant
- a high risk of relapse.

Prevent relapse

The risk of relapse is high for women who, while pregnant and breastfeeding, stop using substances.[3] During pregnancy, the fetus provides daily motivation to abstain from or decrease substance use. Women who have quit

or reduced use need to be re-motivated to deal with the postpartum pressures to return to substance use. Since relapse is often delayed while women are breastfeeding, support for breastfeeding not only provides obvious benefits to the infant, but also presents an opportunity to extend the woman's experience of not using substances post-pregnancy. In this time, providers can help women explore their own intrinsic reasons for cessation.

An example of key principles in action

Sheway is an innovative outreach and drop-in program located in the Downtown Eastside of Vancouver. With a service philosophy that respects and supports women's self-determination in the level and pace of change in their lives, Sheway provides holistic services to pregnant women with substance use problems, and support to mothers and families until their children are 18 months old.

Sheway was established in 1993 in response to a growing understanding of the high levels of substance use by pregnant and parenting women, the low birth weights of their infants and the very high rates of their children's apprehension by child protection authorities. Sheway's services are located in an accessible drop-in setting, and include such key features as:

- practical supports (e.g., hot meals and vitamins, bus tickets, donated clothing and baby equipment, and advocacy on housing and other basic needs)
- health-related and other support by a multidisciplinary team of professionals and paraprofessionals.

Sheway's care providers take a woman-centred, harm reduction–based and culturally focused approach to providing these services.

A 2000 evaluation of Sheway's work brought attention to the difficult lives of pregnant women and new mothers in the Downtown Eastside. It also highlighted the positive role that harm reduction approaches have had in the care of women who use substances and are at high risk, and of their families. The study looked at the outcomes for women who had accessed Sheway's services in 1998, and found that the program had been successful in a number of ways:

- **Engaging women who use substances and are at high risk in prenatal and postnatal care** on a range of health and social issues. At intake, 30 per cent of women had no medical or prenatal care, and by the time of their deliveries 91 per cent of women were connected to a physician or midwife (for the remaining nine per cent, the existence of prenatal and postnatal care was not known).

- **Supporting women as they improve their nutritional status.** Of the women accessing services, 79 per cent had nutritional concerns at intake, whereas only four per cent had nutritional concerns at six months postnatal. (Nutritional concerns were defined as fewer than three meals a day, lack of money to buy adequate food, lack of knowledge of nutrition and food resources [e.g., food banks] or lack of kitchen facilities.) Women who use Sheway's services are provided prenatal vitamins, hot lunches and information about food banks and community kitchens, as well as nutritional counselling—all of which may have contributed to this improvement in nutritional status.

- **Supporting women as they improve their housing.** At intake, 27 per cent of the women had no fixed address, and 65 per cent in total had housing concerns. By six months after the birth of the child, only six per cent of the women had any housing concerns. (Housing concerns were defined as having no housing or having housing of an inadequate size; in a poor location; with overcrowding problems; or with safety, health or structural problems.)

- **Increasing the number of children with healthy birth weights.** Eighty-six per cent of the babies whose mothers accessed care at Sheway were known to have a healthy birth weight (over 2,500 grams).
- **Helping women retain custody of their children.** Over half (58 per cent) of mothers who used Sheway's services were able to retain custody of their children (22 per cent had no involvement by the Ministry for Children and Families, and 36 per cent had ministry involvement for support only). The remaining 42 per cent of mothers did have their children apprehended; in these cases, 37 per cent were later returned to the care of the birth mother or her immediate family.

The evaluation also found that while using Sheway's services, most women had not been able to completely stop using alcohol or other drugs, nor had they been able to participate in intensive substance use treatment. However, Sheway staff have found that stabilization and reduction in substance use are more possible when stability is established in basic life areas such as housing and food security.

Sheway staff, allied service providers and the women themselves see Sheway's service philosophy as critical for women to feel safe and to access the help they need. The positive findings of this 2000 evaluation continue to inform harm reduction–based and woman-centred approaches to work with pregnant women and mothers who use substances and face a range of other health and social problems. In the face of known risks to the health of both mothers and children from substance use and exposure to the dangers of life in Vancouver's Downtown Eastside, Sheway staff continue to expand their practice and understanding of how best to encourage pregnant women with substance use problems to engage in prenatal and postnatal care, and to take realistic, small steps toward change.

Poole, N. (2007). Improving outcomes for women and their children: Evaluation of the Sheway Program. In N. Poole & L. Greaves (Eds.), *Highs & Lows: Canadian Perspectives on Women and Substance Use*. Toronto: Centre for Addiction and Mental Health. Adapted with permission from the *Evaluation Report of the Sheway Project for High-Risk Pregnant and Parenting Women*, authored by Nancy Poole and published in Vancouver by the British Columbia Centre of Excellence for Women's Health in 2000. The full study is available from the centre's website at www.bccewh.bc.ca/ publications-resources/documents/shewayreport.pdf.

References

1. Public Health Agency of Canada. (2004). *The Social Determinants of Health: An Overview of the Implications for Policy and the Role of the Health Sector.* Ottawa: Author. Available: www.phac-aspc. gc.ca/ph-sp/phdd/overview_implications/01_overview.html. Accessed July 13, 2007.

2. Wilkinson, R. & Marmot, M. (2003). *Social Determinants of Health: The Solid Facts* (2nd ed.). Denmark: World Health Organization. Available: www.euro.who.int/document/e81384.pdf. Accessed July 13, 2007.

3. Greaves, L., Cormier, R., Devries, K., Bottorff, J., Johnson, J., Kirkland, S. et al. (2003). *Expecting to Quit: A Best Practices Review of Smoking Cessation Interventions for Pregnant and Postpartum Girls and Women.* Vancouver: British Columbia Centre of Excellence for Women's Health. Available: www.hc-sc.gc.ca/hl-vs/pubs/ tobac-tabac/expecting-grossesse/index_e.html. Accessed July 9, 2007.

4. The "Expecting to Quit" Research Team. (2007). Better practices for smoking cessation with pregnant and postpartum women. In N. Poole & L. Greaves (Eds.), *Highs & Lows: Canadian Perspectives on Women and Substance Use.* Toronto: Centre for Addiction and Mental Health.

5. Statistics Canada. (2003). Canadian Community Health Survey: Mental health and well-being. *The Daily*, September 3. Available: www.statcan.ca/Daily/English/030903/d030903a.htm. Accessed October 5, 2007.

6. Centre for Addiction and Mental Health. (2002). *CAMH Position on Harm Reduction: Its Meaning and Applications For Substance Use Issues.* Toronto: Author. Available: www.camh.net/Public_policy/ Public_policy_papers/publicpolicy_harmreduc2002.html. Accessed July 11, 2007.

7. Adlaf, E.M., Paglia, A. & Beitchman, J.H. (2004). *The Mental Health and Well-Being of Ontario Students: Findings from the OSDUS 1991–2003.* Toronto: Centre for Addiction and Mental Health.

8. Centre for Addiction and Mental Health. (2006). *Navigating Screening Options for Concurrent Disorders.* Toronto: Author.

9. U.S. Department of Health and Human Services. (2002). *A Report to Congress on the Prevention and Treatment of Co-occurring Substance Abuse Disorders and Mental Disorders.* Rockville, MD: Substance Abuse and Mental Health Services Administration.

10. Wise, B.K., Cuffe, S.P. & Fischer, T. (2001). Dual diagnosis and successful participation of adolescents in substance abuse treatment. *Journal of Substance Abuse Treatment, 21* (3), 161–165.

11. Health Canada. (2002). *Best Practices: Concurrent Mental Health and Substance Use Disorders.* Ottawa: Author. Available: www.hc-sc.gc.ca/ahc-asc/pubs/drugs-drogues/index_e.html. Accessed November 1, 2007.

Defining addiction, dependence and abuse

No clear line indicates when substance use becomes a problem that is severe enough to need treatment. However, the fourth edition of the *Diagnostic and Statistical Manual of Mental Disorders* (DSM-IV) includes substance-related disorders as one of the classes of mental disorders. Many clinicians use the DSM-IV's diagnostic criteria for substance abuse and substance dependence to help screen for substance use problems. These criteria are listed on pages 14 to 15.

Addiction versus dependence

The definitions of "addiction" and "dependence" have evolved over the last few decades, and continue to be debated.

Addiction

Addiction is a primary, chronic, neurobiologic disease with genetic, psychosocial and environmental factors that influence its development and manifestations. It is characterized by behaviours that include one or more of the following:

- loss of control over drug use
- continued use despite harm
- compulsive use and craving.

There are several theories of addiction, but the most compelling one views it as a multifactorial disease caused by predisposing and precipitating factors.[2] This view

The four Cs of addiction[1]

FEATURE	TYPICAL STATEMENTS
Loss of **C**ontrol over use	"Every time I try to limit my use to only once a week, I end up using every day."
	"I try to limit myself to one drink per day but once I start, I can't seem to stop until I pass out."
Continued use despite knowledge of harmful **C**onsequences	"I know my drug use caused my HIV but I can't stop using."
	"I have to stop using because my life is out of control, but using is the only option for me."
Compulsion to use	"All I do is think about how I am going to score."
	"No matter what I do, I can't get drugs out of my mind and I feel I have to use and use a lot. Once I want to use, it is like I am on autopilot and I just have to use. I'll do anything to get drugs."
Craving	"It's like a physical drive or urge to use. I want it from the pit of my stomach; I get sweaty just thinking about it. At times, these urges come out of nowhere, or I get them when I meet my using buddies, pass the corner where my dealer hangs out or am feeling down."

Exposure to Psychotropic Medications and Other Substances during Pregnancy and Lactation

describes the disease as the interaction between host (i.e., the person who is addicted to the substance), agent (i.e., the drug) and environmental determinants (i.e., social determinants of health), affected by a vector (e.g., a person or an industry that promotes the drug and/or creates conducive conditions for its increased use and the subsequent harm associated with that use).[3] And there is emerging evidence that the neurobiology of addiction provides the basis for understanding why people have great difficulty remaining abstinent, even years after withdrawal is overcome.[4–6]

Physical dependence

Physical dependence is often thought to be the thing that defines addiction, but this is not always necessary or sufficient for a diagnosis of substance dependence. Nevertheless, understanding the components of physical dependence is important because discontinuation of some substances requires clinical management. The two related observable phenomena that comprise physical dependence are tolerance and withdrawal.

TOLERANCE

Tolerance is due to compensatory changes, such as downregulation and desensitization, in the number and sensitivity of central nervous system receptors. Over time, these changes compel a person to take more of the drug to achieve the same effect; or if the person maintains the same level and pattern of consumption, she stops experiencing the desired effect. The time it takes to develop tolerance to the various effects of a given drug differs considerably.

WITHDRAWAL

Withdrawal is a specific syndrome that often begins within a few hours of stopping a drug. This occurs because the downregulation of receptors leads to unstable neurotransmission. These receptors take days or weeks to normalize with abstinence, creating a constellation of symptoms and signs that are opposite to the drug's main effect.

The acute withdrawal for most drugs starts within a half-life of the drug, peaks within three to five half-lives of the drug and then resolves within a week or two at most; however, this is often followed by intense cravings for the drug, dysphoric mood and other symptoms that can lead to relapse.

Substance-related disorders

The DSM-IV-TR[7] classifies substance-related disorders as substance use disorders (which are further categorized as either substance dependence and substance abuse) or substance-induced disorders. The criteria for substance use disorders follow.

DSM-IV-TR criteria for substance dependence

A maladaptive pattern of substance use, leading to clinically significant impairment or distress, as manifested by three (or more) of the following, occurring at any time in the same 12-month period:

1. *tolerance, as defined by either of the following:*
   a. *a need for markedly increased amounts of the substance to achieve intoxication or desired effect*
   b. *markedly diminished effect with continued use of the same amount of the substance*
2. *withdrawal, as manifested by either of the following:*
   a. *the characteristic withdrawal syndrome for the substance . . .*
   b. *the same (or a closely related) substance is taken to relieve or avoid withdrawal symptoms*
3. *the substance is often taken in larger amounts or over a longer period than was intended*
4. *there is a persistent desire or [there are] unsuccessful efforts to cut down or control substance use*
5. *a great deal of time is spent in activities necessary to obtain the substance (e.g., visiting multiple doctors or driving long distances), use the substance (e.g., chain smoking), or recover from its effects*
6. *important social, occupational, or recreational activities are given up or reduced because of substance use*
7. *the substance use is continued despite knowledge of having a persistent or recurrent physical or psychological problem that is likely to have been caused or exacerbated by the substance (e.g., current cocaine use despite recognition of cocaine-induced depression, or continued drinking despite recognition that an ulcer was made worse by alcohol consumption).*

DSM-IV-TR criteria for substance abuse

A. *A maladaptive pattern of substance use leading to clinically significant impairment or distress, as manifested by one (or more) of the following, occurring within a 12-month period:*

1. *recurrent substance use resulting in a failure to fulfil major role obligations at work, school, or home (e.g., repeated absences or poor work performance related to substance use; substance-related absences, suspensions, or expulsions from school; neglect of children or household)*
2. *recurrent substance use in situations in which it is physically hazardous (e.g., driving an automobile or operating a machine when impaired by substance use)*
3. *recurrent substance-related legal problems (e.g., arrests for substance-related disorderly conduct)*

4. continued substance use despite having persistent or recurrent social or interpersonal problems caused or exacerbated by the effects of the substance (e.g., arguments with spouse about consequences of intoxication, physical fights)

B. The symptoms have never met the criteria for substance dependence for this class of substance. *

References

1. Graham, A.W., Schultz, T.K., Mayo-Smith, M.F., Ries, R.K. & Wilford, B.B. (Eds.). (2003). *Principles of Addiction Medicine* (3rd ed.). Washington, DC: American Society of Addiction Medicine.

2. Volkow, N.D. & Li, T.K. (2005). Drugs and alcohol: Treating and preventing abuse, addiction and their medical consequences. *Pharmacology and Therapeutics, 108* (1), 3–17.

3. Volkow, N.D. (2005). What do we know about drug addiction? *American Journal of Psychiatry, 162* (8), 1401–1402.

4. Hyman, S.E. (2005). Addiction: A disease of learning and memory. *American Journal of Psychiatry, 162* (8), 1414–1422.

5. Hyman, S.E. & Malenka, R.C. (2001). Addiction and the brain: The neurobiology of compulsion and its persistence. *Nature Reviews: Neuroscience, 2* (10), 695–703.

6. Hyman, S.E., Malenka, R.C. & Nestler, E.J. (2006). Neural mechanisms of addiction: The role of reward-related learning and memory. *Annual Review of Neuroscience, 29,* 565–598.

7. American Psychiatric Association. (2000). *Diagnostic and Statistical Manual of Mental Disorders* (4th ed., text rev.). Washington, DC: Author.

* Reprinted with permission from the *Diagnostic and Statistical Manual of Mental Disorders*, Fourth Edition, Text Revision. Copyright 2000. American Psychiatric Association.

Screening

Screening and assessment are often spoken of as one process. While they often overlap, there are significant differences between the two. *Screening* uses simple, brief procedures, often no more than a list of standard questions, to determine whether a person is likely to have a substance use problem. If a problem is likely, *assessment* uses more in-depth and ongoing processes to identify substance-related disorders.

Screening can be done by phone or face-to-face. The screening method can be tailored to clients' needs and to the needs of the health care setting. Other considerations include using questions that are appropriate for the age, culture and literacy level of a client.

Screening for alcohol, tobacco, illegal drug and psychotropic medication use should be undertaken with all pregnant women and, for planned pregnancies, can begin during a preconception visit. As part of the overall health examination, women should be asked about their use of psychotropic medication and other drugs during each trimester, and again after delivery. Asking screening questions can lead to an open discussion about alcohol, tobacco and other drug use. In talking with women about problematic medication and substance use during pregnancy, health care providers can determine appropriate interventions in a timely fashion, which may help improve both the mother's and the baby's health outcomes.

Screening questions, rather than drug toxicology tests alone, continue to be the most effective method for detecting those at risk for alcohol or other drug problems. Toxicology tests are based on detecting particular drug concentrations at a certain point in time, and so may miss substance use if the test does not coincide with a drug's detection period. To engage women in addiction treatment, it is ideal that screening for those at risk of substance use problems be based on self-report. During screening, a provider follows general questions with more specific ones which are chosen depending upon the woman's responses.

A variety of screening questionnaires have been developed to detect substance use in pregnancy. They are brief, easily administered and readily incorporated into routine prenatal care.

Prevalence studies have found that the following characteristics are usually present in women at higher risk of substance use during pregnancy:[2,3]

- polysubstance abuse (i.e., concurrent abuse of more than one psychotropic medication and/or illegal substance)
- low socio-economic status
- less formal education
- stressful life events

lack of a supportive social network (e.g., being without a caring and helpful partner or living with a partner or household member who uses drugs)

history of mental health disorders (e.g., mood, anxiety or eating disorders)

history of physical or sexual abuse

family history of substance abuse

lack of adequate prenatal care.

However, women who are older and have higher socio-economic status and higher levels of education have also been found to have higher rates of alcohol use in pregnancy, and so are a special population to be considered.[4] This is one of the reasons why universal screening is so important.

General screening questions

Screening tools can help identify women who are at risk for problematic substance use and who may need more in-depth assessment by a primary care provider such as a family physician or nurse practitioner, or a health care specialist such as an obstetrician, a psychiatrist or an addiction medicine professional.[1] Ideally, screening questions are introduced as a normal part of any visit with a health care provider; the rationale for such a discussion can be explained within the context of the woman's overall health status.

Building trust and rapport with the woman is critical to screening for problematic substance use,[1,2] as is a non-judgmental approach to both negative substance use disclosures (i.e., that a woman is not using) and positive substance use disclosures (i.e., that a woman is using). A woman may deny any drug use when asked the first time but, depending on the quality of the client-provider relationship and the way that she was initially asked about her substance use, may acknowledge use on subsequent questioning.

Health care providers are advised to encourage dialogue with a woman by initially asking open-ended questions, which can feel less intrusive, about less sensitive areas (e.g., medications) before proceeding to questions related to illegal drugs. Then the focus can shift to areas where a woman has reported problematic substance use.

The questions on the following pages, which have been adapted from multiple toolkits, are examples of ways to approach the subject of substance use with pregnant and breastfeeding women. Health care providers need to ask questions sensitively but directly.

The majority of research on physician performance in the area of substance use—which has largely focused on alcohol problems—suggests that "physicians perform poorly in screening and counselling patients with alcohol problems. . . . Physicians commonly report that lack of knowledge and training is a barrier to their detection and management of substance use"[5] (pp. 1–2). Clinicians may be uncomfortable asking questions about an area where they lack clinical expertise. A health care provider who is not comfortable asking questions about substance use needs to learn to, or find support to, increase his or her comfort level, because these questions are an important part of providing overall health care. Providers can phrase the questions in their own words to fit their own comfort level; the more often they ask these questions, the more comfortable they will become with them. In addition, it is important for providers to be aware of community resources and agencies so they can refer women for the support and information they need.

Screening questions about psychotropic drug use

"Do you use any prescription medications to help with mental health symptoms, such as mood and anxiety symptoms?"

If the woman answers "yes"	→ Ask about the source of the medication and how the woman is using it (e.g., ask: "Did your doctor write you a prescription for this medication, or did you get it from another place?" If it is a prescribed medication, ask: "Are you following the directions on the prescription or using the medication differently?")
	→ Ask about the pattern (amount and frequency) of medication use (e.g., ask: "How much are you taking and how often are you taking it?")
	→ Assess the stage of change (see Figure 2 on page 21) the woman may be at with respect to problematic psychotropic drug use (e.g., ask: "How do you feel about making a change in your medication use?")

Screening questions about alcohol use[3]

"How much alcohol do you drink?"

If the woman indicates that she drinks alcohol	→ Ask about the pattern (amount and frequency) of use, and about any binge drinking—heavy episodic drinking, during which a person consumes five or more standard drinks on one occasion (e.g., ask: "In a typical week, on how many days do you drink? On those days, how many drinks would you usually have?")
	→ Assess the stage of change the woman may be at with respect to alcohol use (e.g., ask: "How do you feel about stopping drinking?")
	(These questions can be followed by the T-ACE or TWEAK questionnaires, on pages 23 and 24, to detect at-risk drinking.)
If the woman indicates that she does not drink alcohol	→ Determine any prenatal exposure to alcohol during the early part of the pregnancy (e.g., ask: "Before you knew that you were pregnant, did you drink alcohol?")

Screening questions about tobacco use[6,7]

"Do you smoke?"

If the woman answers "yes"	→ Ask about the pattern (amount and duration) of tobacco use (e.g., ask: "How much do you smoke and how long have you smoked?")
	→ Assess the stage of change the woman may be at with respect to smoking cessation (e.g., ask: "How do you feel about quitting smoking?")
If the woman answers "no"	→ Screen for second-hand smoke exposure (e.g., ask: "Does anyone smoke around you or your children?")

Screening questions about illegal drug use

"Have you ever used cannabis, cocaine or any other recreational drugs?"

If the woman answers "yes"	→ Enquire about the kind of drug (e.g., ask: "What drug(s) do you use currently?")
	→ Ask about the pattern (amount and frequency) of illegal drug use (e.g., ask: "How much are you using and how often?")
	→ Assess the stage of change the woman may be at with respect to illegal drug use (e.g., ask: "How do you feel about stopping your use of illegal drugs?")
If the woman answers "no"	→ Determine any history of illegal drug use before the pregnancy (e.g., ask: "Have you used illegal drugs in the past?")
	→ Ask about any drug use during an earlier part of this pregnancy (e.g., ask: "Have you ever used illegal drugs during this pregnancy?")
	→ Screen for exposure to drugs in the woman's/child's environment (e.g., ask: "Does anyone use illegal drugs around you or your child?")

Figure 2: Stages of change

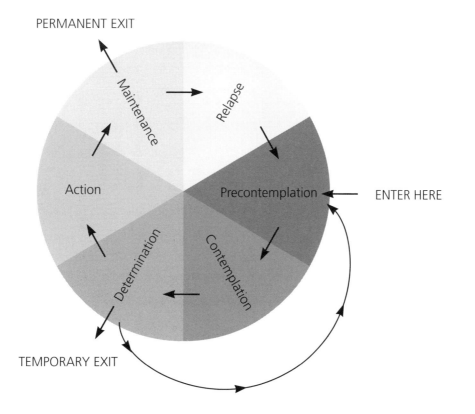

Adapted from Prochaska, J.O. & DiClemente, C.C. (1982). Transtheoretical therapy: Toward a more integrative model of change. *Psychotherapy: Theory, Research and Practice, 19* (3), 276–288.

Screening questionnaires

The Antenatal Psychosocial Health Assessment (ALPHA) form, the T-ACE and the TWEAK have been developed and validated for use with pregnant women.[8–12] These instruments (discussed below) are easily incorporated into a provider-client interview. Both the T-ACE and TWEAK have been shown to be highly sensitive in the detection of periconceptional risk drinking. A positive screen indicates the need for further assessment of alcohol use by the pregnant woman. (*Risk drinking* during pregnancy is defined as the level of maternal alcohol consumption associated with adverse outcomes [i.e., one ounce or more of absolute alcohol per day, the equivalent of two or more drinks per day, or 14 or more drinks per week].)

Antenatal Psychosocial Health Assessment form

To ensure that psychosocial assessment becomes a routine part of prenatal care, the University of Toronto's Faculty of Medicine developed the ALPHA form after a comprehensive literature review.[12] This guide addresses four categories of factors:

- family factors (e.g., social support, stressful life events, relationship with partner)

- maternal factors (e.g., prenatal care, prenatal education, feelings toward pregnancy, relationship with parents during childhood, self-esteem, history of mental health problems, depression in current pregnancy)
- substance use (e.g., alcohol and other drug abuse, partner's substance use)
- family violence (e.g., experiencing or witnessing physical, emotional or sexual abuse; experience of and thoughts about child discipline).

Problems identified in these areas have been associated with poor postpartum outcomes such as child and woman abuse, couple dysfunction, postpartum depression and increased infant physical illness.

The substance use section of the form enquires about alcohol and other drug use during pregnancy through a series of general screening questions, followed by the CAGE questionnaire (see next page).

Two versions of the ALPHA form are available: a provider-completed form and a patient self-report. (Links to English and French versions of the ALPHA forms can be accessed at http://dfcm.utoronto.ca/research/alpha/.)

CAGE

The CAGE screening questionnaire is incorporated into the ALPHA form as a screen for problematic alcohol use.[13] However, this tool is adaptable to asking about other drug use as well.

C	Cut down	Have you ever felt you should cut down on your drinking?
A	Annoyed	Have people annoyed you by criticizing your drinking?
G	Guilty	Have you felt guilty about your drinking?
E	Eye-opener	Have you ever had a drink first thing in the morning to steady your nerves or get rid of a hangover?

Scoring: Each yes response equals a score of 1. A total score of 1 may indicate the need for further discussion. A total score of 2 or greater is clinically significant, suggesting current or past alcohol problem and, therefore, warranting more in-depth assessment.

T-ACE

The T-ACE questionnaire has been extensively validated in different obstetrical populations.[8,9] It has been shown to be effective as a self-administered screening tool and a one-minute screen used by practitioners as part of routine care. T-ACE has a sensitivity* of 70 per cent and a specificity† of 85 per cent.

T	Tolerance	How many drinks does it take for you to feel high?
A	Annoyed	Have people annoyed you by criticizing your drinking?
C	Cut down	Have you ever felt you should cut down on your drinking?
E	Eye-opener	Have you ever had a drink first thing in the morning to steady your nerves or get rid of a hangover?

Scoring: Any woman who answers the tolerance question by indicating that she needs more than two drinks is scored 2 points. Each yes response to the additional three questions receives a score of 1. A score of 2 or more indicates risk of a drinking problem, and the woman should be considered for further assessment.

*Correct identification of people who meet the criteria for a particular diagnosis or problem.
†Correct identification of people who do not meet the criteria for a particular diagnosis or problem.

TWEAK

The TWEAK questionnaire has also been shown to be effective at detecting risk drinking among pregnant women.[10,11] This questionnaire has no advantages over T-ACE but is an alternative method for screening for alcohol use. TWEAK has a sensitivity of 79 per cent and a specificity of 83 per cent.

T	Tolerance	How many drinks does it take for you to feel high?
W	Worries	Do family members or friends ever worry or complain about your drinking?
E	Eye-opener	Have you ever had a drink first thing in the morning to steady your nerves or get rid of a hangover?
A	Amnesia/ blackouts	Have you ever awakened the morning after drinking the night before and found that you could not remember part of the evening?
K	K/Cut down	Have you ever felt that you should cut down on your drinking?

Scoring: A woman receives 2 points on the tolerance question if she reports that she needs three or more drinks to feel the effect of alcohol. A positive response to the worry question scores 2 points. A positive response to each of the last three questions scores 1 point each. A total score of 2 or more indicates that the woman is a risk drinker and requires further assessment.

References

1. Morse, B., Gehshan, S. & Hutchins, E. (1997). *Screening for Substance Abuse during Pregnancy: Improving Care, Improving Health.* Arlington, VA: National Center for Education in Maternal and Child Health.

2. Gavin, K. (2003). *The Help Guide for Professionals Working with Women Who Use Substances.* Edmonton: Alberta Alcohol and Drug Abuse Commission.

3. Best Start. (2002). *Supporting Change: Preventing and Addressing Alcohol Use in Pregnancy.* Toronto: Ontario Prevention Clearing House.

4. Dzakpasu, S., Mery, L.S. & Trouton, K. (1998). *Canadian Perinatal Surveillance System: Alcohol and Pregnancy.* Ottawa: Health Canada.

5. Kahan, M., Midmer, D., Wilson, L. & Borsoi, D. (2007). Medical students' knowledge about alcohol and drug problems: Results of the Medical Council of Canada Examination. *Substance Abuse: Journal of the Association for Medical Education and Research in Substance Abuse, 27* (4), 1–7.

6. Greaves, L., Cormier, R., Devries, K., Bottorff, J., Johnson, J., Kirkland, S. et al. (2003). *Expecting to Quit: A Best Practices Review of Smoking Cessation Interventions for Pregnant and Postpartum Girls and Women.* Vancouver: British Columbia Centre of Excellence for Women's Health. Available: www.hc-sc.gc.ca/hl-vs/pubs/tobac-tabac/expecting-grossesse/index_e.html. Accessed July 13, 2007.

7. Pregnets. (2005). *Smoking Cessation during Pregnancy.* Available: www.pregnets.org/providers/downloads.aspx. Accessed July 13, 2007.

8. Sokol, R.J., Martier, S.S. & Ager, J.W. (1989). The T-ACE questions: Practical prenatal detection of risk drinking. *American Journal of Obstetrics and Gynecology, 160* (4), 863–870.

9. Russell, M., Martier, S.S., Sokol, R.J., Mudar, P., Jacobson, S. & Jacobson, J. (1996). Detecting risk drinking during pregnancy: A comparison of four screening questionnaires. *American Journal of Public Health, 86* (10), 1435–1439.

10. Russell, M. (1994). New assessment tools for risk drinking during pregnancy: T-ACE, TWEAK, and others. *Alcohol Health and Research World, 18* (1), 55–61.

11. Chang, G., Wilkins-Haug, L., Berman, S. & Goetz, M.A. (1999). The TWEAK: Application in a prenatal setting. *Journal of Studies on Alcohol, 60* (3), 306–309.

12. Midmer, D., Biringer, A., Carroll, J.C., Reid, A.J., Wilson, L., Stewart, D. et al. (1996). *A Reference Guide for Providers: The ALPHA Form—Antenatal Psychosocial Health Assessment Form.* (2nd ed.). Toronto: University of Toronto.

13. Mayfield, D., McLeod, G. & Hall, P. (1974). The CAGE questionnaire: Validation of a new alcoholism screening instrument. *American Journal of Psychiatry, 131* (10), 1121–1123.

The therapeutic relationship

Factors in recovery

Even without specific training as a counsellor, health care practitioners who provide care to pregnant women with substance use and/or mental health problems can play a key therapeutic role in helping women move toward a better health outcome. Listening to women's concerns and fears, and offering guidance and reassurance, can help providers be effective health care allies. Stigma and marginalization prevent many women with substance use and mental health problems from presenting to health care providers. Even women who do enter prenatal care are likely to feel guarded and ashamed of their substance use and/or mental illness. Understanding stigma's effects and responding non-judgmentally to women who are reluctant to participate in care may help women become more engaged in their own treatment process.

Research confirms that a positive therapeutic relationship between a provider and a client has a helpful impact. Michael Lambert has explored factors that lead to successful change in someone's life (see Figure 3). Lambert[1] concluded that:

- 40 per cent of a client's ability to manifest positive change is attributable to extra-therapeutic factors (e.g., safe and stable housing, secure employment, adequate financial resources, positive interactions, supports in the community)

- 30 per cent is attributable to a client's experience of the therapeutic relationship (e.g., a health care provider's non-judgmental attitude, warmth, respect and caring)

- 15 per cent is attributable to a client's sense of hope and expectation for recovery

- 15 per cent is attributable to the provider's techniques and skills (e.g., cognitive-behavioural therapy, mindfulness-based stress reduction).

Figure 3: Factors influencing ability to change

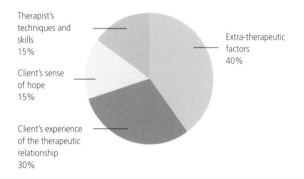

Therapist's techniques and skills 15%

Client's sense of hope 15%

Client's experience of the therapeutic relationship 30%

Extra-therapeutic factors 40%

Therefore, health care providers can have a significant impact by helping a woman find adequate housing and work and develop stable, positive interactions in her life outside of therapy; by focusing on the quality of the therapeutic relationship; by using appropriate therapeutic techniques and skills; and by fostering her sense of hope or change. Encouraging a sense of optimism greatly enhances other factors, such as the therapeutic relationship, and is key to influencing a person's ability to change.

Communication

A health care provider's communication style can affect how a woman responds to his or her advice. Even subtle perceived negative attitudes can undermine a woman's trust in her provider. Care in a provider's choice of words, demeanour and attention can make it easier for a woman to listen and communicate, and to act on new knowledge.

Using good communication skills includes:

    showing empathy through engaging in reflective listening (See "Motivational Interviewing" on page 28)

    creating a safe space where a woman can ask any question and disclose medication or other substance use

    clearly explaining a woman's options

    focusing on a woman's strengths

    asking open-ended questions

    using clear language

    providing feedback

    taking a non-judgmental approach

    inviting a woman to share her point of view or concerns.

In addition to general communications skills, it is critical for a provider to be prepared to answer difficult questions, for example: "Will child protection services take my baby away?" "What happens if I test positive after giving birth?" "What happens if my baby goes into withdrawal?" "Do you have to tell my partner about the things we talk about?" "Will you report me if I tell you something in confidence?" It is important to respond directly and immediately to women's questions, to provide specific information and to be clear and upfront. Women who ask tough questions but don't get "straight answers" from their health care providers often become guarded and uncertain about disclosing information.

Health care providers may see a woman several times over the course of her pregnancy, and any contact is also an opportunity to develop a trusting relationship with her. During clinical appointments, providers can explore:

• a woman's behaviours (e.g., has she been using more, the same amount, less, or has she stopped using altogether? how has she been coping with using or not using? what has been challenging or positive about what she has been doing?)

• the risks and safety of medications and other substances

• whether a woman has appropriate support, such as a caring and encouraging partner, family member or friend (since stigma can make a woman feel that she isn't worthy of support, it is important to validate her right to it)

- whether she faces issues such as poverty, trauma or racism, or inaccessible environments that exacerbate the challenges a disability presents—and, if so, how she feels these issues impact her life and how she deals with them
- whether she has experienced or is currently experiencing violence and/or abuse
- how she copes with conflict and difficult emotions (research[2] has shown that women are at highest risk for using substances when they feel negative emotions and experience conflict with others)
- how she feels about taking medication
- how she feels about using other substances (e.g., does she feel that using substances harms her? does she feel that it helps her with something such as distracting her from painful memories of abuse?)
- what she knows about the impact of her substance use on her health and the health of her fetus or infant
- whether she would like more information about the impact of her substance use on her fetus or infant, and/or whether she has been misled by myths and misinformation

- how she feels about her pregnancy
- whether she has envisioned and/or has planned for her life after her child is born (e.g., whether she will have parenting and childcare support, whether she will have safe housing, whether she will be financially secure).

Overall, use of good communication skills can help motivate clients toward positive behavioural change, help them stay actively engaged in their own care and instil hope for the future.

Motivational interviewing

The most common definition of motivational interviewing is a "client-centered, directive method for enhancing intrinsic motivation to change by exploring and resolving ambivalence"[3] (p. 25). The word "interviewing," rather than "counselling" or "treatment," stresses the egalitarian nature of the encounter between provider and client and the fact that they are "viewing" things together.[3]

Motivational interviewing has been shown to be particularly helpful in working with people who use substances.[4] This method focuses on clients' experiences; draws on their concerns, perspectives and values; and encourages clients to evaluate their own life choices and explore the consequences of their choices in a non-judgmental way.

Four principles guide motivational interviewing:

expressing empathy

developing discrepancy

rolling with resistance

supporting self-efficacy.

Expressing empathy

Motivational interviewing uses an empathic communication style. This is achieved through the therapeutic skill of reflective listening.

REFLECTIVE LISTENING

When listening reflectively, the counsellor mirrors, in his or her own words, what the client says and checks that he or she correctly understood the client. As the provider asks open-ended questions and reflects back the client's words, feelings, context and experience in a respectful and non-judgmental manner, the client comes to feel understood and accepted. Paradoxically, when people feel accepted as they are, they become freer to change than when they are told they need to change. The counsellor sees ambivalence about changing as a normal part of the process.[3] Reflective listening is also key to building the client-counsellor relationship, in that it conveys empathy, understanding and acceptance.

Reflective listening is difficult to master, and providers may unwittingly set up roadblocks that can prevent clients from exploring or elaborating on a problem or issue. Some of these roadblocks may even trigger or intensify resistance to change. These roadblocks[3] (p. 68) include:

- acting as the expert

- giving advice, making suggestions or providing solutions without first listening to the client's ideas and asking permission

- questioning or probing in areas that the client does not see as relevant

- ordering, directing or commanding

- warning or threatening

- disagreeing, arguing or lecturing

- judging, criticizing, moralizing, labelling, shaming, ridiculing or blaming

- agreeing, approving or praising—not to be confused with statements of affirmation

- withdrawing, distracting, humouring or changing the subject.

There are several levels of reflective listening. The most simplistic is to parrot or echo, virtually word for word, what a client says. More complex reflective listening conveys deeper reflection of the client's meaning, including mirroring the emotional aspect of a client's words and linking those feelings to her expressed thoughts and to life events.

Developing discrepancy

An important way to help a woman resolve ambivalence is to highlight and amplify discrepancies, from her perspective, between the present behaviour and broader goals and values. Change can be triggered by her heightened awareness that a current behaviour is getting in the way of achieving important goals, or that it conflicts with important values. Discrepancies provide reasons to change. Developing discrepancy involves exploring how she would like to see herself, and how the current behaviour conflicts with that vision. By becoming aware of discrepancies, she can find and articulate her own reasons for changing, rather than having the provider give reasons for change.[3]

Rolling with resistance

In motivational interviewing, the counsellor avoids confrontation and does not directly oppose a client's resistance to change. Arguing for change—or even taking up the side of the client's ambivalence that favours change—usually leads to a counterproductive dynamic in which clients feel they have to defend their position and they become entrenched in resistance. Instead, the counsellor views resistance as a natural part of change and uses it as an opportunity to involve the client in weighing the pros and cons of continuing behaviours and exploring options for and barriers to change. Respecting that a woman is the primary resource for finding answers and solutions, the provider invites—but does not impose—new perspectives. How the provider responds to resistance will influence whether it increases or decreases; resistance is a sign for the provider to shift his or her approach and a cue to examine the woman's underlying assumptions about change.[3]

Supporting self-efficacy

Self-efficacy refers to a person's belief that she has the ability to carry out, and succeed at, a specific task. For change to occur, a woman must have a sense that change is possible and that she can make it happen—the sense of expectancy and hope for recovery is noted in Figure 3 on page 26. To build her self-confidence, the counsellor can explore the woman's past successes, or provide successful role models that she can identify with.[3] The provider's belief in the woman's ability to change is key, but the woman, not the provider, is responsible for choosing and carrying out change.

Trauma and safety

A crucial determinant of maternal and fetal health involves assessing a woman for current violence, safety or trauma issues and providing immediate resources if issues arise. Many women who struggle with substance use and mental health issues have experienced sexual or physical abuse in their past. For example, as much as 38 per cent of the general population in Ontario report childhood physical or sexual abuse.[5] And in a U.S. national comorbidity study,[6] which surveyed a sample of adults in the general population, the estimated lifetime exposure to severe traumatic events was 61 per cent in men and 51 per cent in women. Women were more likely than men to develop stress symptoms following rape, sexual molestation and physical attack, being threatened with a weapon or childhood physical abuse. While men were more likely than women to be exposed to traumatic conditions, women were twice as likely to develop symptoms of posttraumatic stress disorder (10 per cent vs. five per cent). This difference may be related to the fact that women are 13 times more likely than men to be raped or sexually molested.[6]

A 2000 report states that:

Among those seeking help for substance use problems, women report past abuse much more frequently than men. In fact, most women in substance use treatment programs report physical and sexual abuse over their lifetime, and about one-quarter have received a diagnosis of post-traumatic stress disorder (PTSD).[7] (p. 416)

In addition, research suggests that when women involved in violent or abusive relationships become pregnant, the violence and abuse often continue during the pregnancy, although in some situations abuse may begin when a woman becomes pregnant.[8] Up to 40 per cent of first incidents of domestic violence occur while the woman is pregnant.[9]

Supportive discussions at every visit can help reassure a woman that she has choices and options in terms of dealing with violence and trauma. Connecting her with supports (e.g., agencies, services) can help her cope with these issues as well as the physical and emotional challenges of pregnancy.

Legal issues

Health care providers in Canada have a legal responsibility to report any child who needs or may need child protection services; this obligation only applies to the child once born. Providers should contact their local child protection services for reporting responsibilities and procedures, and should discuss the issue and obtain written consent from the pregnant woman if considering a referral to a child protection service during the prenatal period.

Many women who use substances fear their provider will report them to authorities, which presents a challenge in attending to their health care needs. Helping a woman understand her rights and the provider's responsibilities—before the birth—can help her to make decisions around her substance use while pregnant and to evaluate her behaviour. Women should be encouraged to have open communication with child protection services. Decisions regarding supervision and custody are less likely to be adversarial when women are engaged in services.[10] (See "An Example of Key Principles in Action" on pages 8 to 10 for an illustration of an outreach program that has successfully worked with child protection services and women who use substances to help women retain custody of their children.)

It may also be helpful for care providers to introduce the woman to the supportive services (e.g., parenting classes) available through child protection services before the child is born. This would provide further opportunities for her to discuss her concerns (e.g., how she would be followed clinically; whether she would be able to take her child home; what the expectations for behaviour change would be in order to regain custody and access, if the child were removed from her care).

If a woman presents to a provider with probable signs of violence, a health care provider will have to decide whether it might be appropriate to contact other agencies or authorities to help protect the woman. It is important to consult with a woman's advocacy service such as a rape crisis centre or a legal clinic to get clarification about what can and cannot be disclosed about potential abuse a woman may face, and about the roles and limits of police and court powers.

Summary

Developing trust and rapport with a woman becomes more feasible when a provider shows empathy, communicates well, has a thorough grasp of the realities of the woman's life, draws on effective counselling strategies, uses a non-judgmental approach and understands the legal issues regarding the safety of the woman and her baby. Being able to talk comfortably and sensitively—but also directly—about difficult and "taboo" subjects such as substance use encourages open dialogue and honesty, which can lead the woman to become more fully informed and in a better position to make optimal choices for both her own and her child's well-being.

References

1. Lambert, M.J., Implications of outcome research for psychotherapy integration. In Norcross, J.C. & Goldstein, M.R., *Handbook of Psychotherapy Intergration* (pp. 94–129). New York: Basic Books. Cited in Centre for Addiction and Mental Health. (2005). *Beyond the Label: An Educational Kit to Promote Awareness and Understanding of the Impact of Stigma on People Living with Concurrent Mental Health and Substance Use Problems.* Toronto: Author. Available: www.camh.net/About_Addiction_Mental_Health/ Concurrent_Disorders/beyond_the_label_toolkit05.pdf. Accessed July 13, 2007.

2. Harrison, S. & Ingber, E. (2004). Working with women. In S. Harrison & V. Carver (Eds.), *Alcohol & Drug Problems: A Practical Guide for Counsellors* (3rd ed.; pp. 247–271). Toronto: Centre for Addiction and Mental Health.

3. Miller, W.R. & Rollnick, S. (2002). *Motivational Interviewing: Preparing People for Change* (2nd ed.). New York: Guilford Press.

4. Burke, B.L., Arkowitz, H. & Dunn, C. (2002). The efficacy of motivational interviewing and its adaptations: What we know so far. In W.R. Miller & S. Rollnick (Eds.), *Motivational Interviewing: Preparing People for Change* (2nd ed.). New York: Guilford Press.

5. MacMillan, H.L., Fleming, J.E., Trocmé, N., Boyle, M.H., Wong, M., Racine, Y.A. et al. (1997). Prevalence of child physical and sexual abuse in the community: Results from the Ontario Health Supplement. *Journal of the American Medical Association, 278* (2), 131–135. Cited in Gitberg, M. & Van Wyk, L. (2004). Trauma and substance use. In S. Harrison & V. Carver (Eds.), *Alcohol & Drug Problems: A Practical Guide for Counsellors* (3rd ed.; pp. 415–434). Toronto: Centre for Addiction and Mental Health.

6. Chu, J.A. (1998). *Rebuilding Shattered Lives: The Responsible Treatment of Complex Post-traumatic and Dissociative Disorders.* New York: John Wiley & Sons. Cited in Gitberg, M. & Van Wyk, L. (2004). Trauma and substance use. In S. Harrison & V. Carver (Eds.), *Alcohol & Drug Problems: A Practical Guide for Counsellors* (3rd ed.; pp. 415–434). Toronto: Centre for Addiction and Mental Health.

7. Ouimette, P.C., Kimmerling, R., Shaw, J. & Moos, R.H. (2000). Physical and sexual abuse among men and women with substance use disorders. *Alcoholism Treatment Quarterly, 18* (3), 7–17. Cited in Gitberg, M. & Van Wyk, L. (2004). Trauma and substance use. In S. Harrison & V. Carver (Eds.), *Alcohol & Drug Problems: A Practical Guide for Counsellors* (3rd ed.; pp. 415–434). Toronto: Centre for Addiction and Mental Health.

8. Public Health Agency of Canada. (2004). Physical Abuse during Pregnancy. Available: www.phac-aspc.gc.ca/rhs-ssg/factshts/ abuseprg_e.html. Accessed July 8, 2007.

9. Rodgers, K. (1994). Wife assault: The findings of a national survey. *Juristat, 14* (9), 1–21. Cited in Greaves, L., Cormier, R., Devries, K., Bottorff, J., Johnson, J., Kirkland, S. et al. (2003), *Expecting to Quit: A Best Practices Review of Smoking Cessation Interventions for Pregnant and Postpartum Girls and Women.* Vancouver: British Columbia Centre of Excellence for Women's Health. Available: www.hc-sc.gc.ca/hl-vs/pubs/tobac-tabac/expecting-grossesse/ index_e.html. Accessed July 9, 2007.

10. Selby, P. & Ordean, A. (2007). Hospitals, doctors and pregnant women with substance use problems: Working together. In N. Poole and L. Greaves (Eds.), *Highs & Lows: Canadian Perspectives on Women and Substance Use.* Toronto: Centre for Addiction and Mental Health.

Psychotropic Medications and Other Substances

PROPERTIES, EFFECTS AND RECOMMENDATIONS

Introductory issues

Ideally, all pregnancies would be planned, in order to ensure that a woman feels positive about her pregnancy and has the support and resources she needs to care for herself and her child. Planned pregnancies also help to ensure that the fetus is not exposed to harmful substances that may cause adverse effects. However, it is well known that 50 per cent of all pregnancies are unplanned.[1] Consequently a fetus may be exposed to harmful substances that a woman would not have taken had she known she was pregnant.

While current research suggests that some illegal drugs pose less of a direct harm to a fetus or infant than originally thought, these results should be seen as neither an endorsement of the safety of these substances nor an endorsement of their use. Associated environmental factors (e.g., child neglect, poor nutrition, criminal activity, unsafe housing) contribute to an unhealthy and potentially harmful environment.

The mental health of a mother is key to the health of her baby. Women are often told—by well-meaning friends and family, the media and even health care providers—to stop taking psychiatric medications in pregnancy, and/or to choose between breastfeeding or their medication. However, this advice does not take into account the negative effects that untreated illness or abrupt withdrawal can have on both the mother and the baby. In fact, the American Academy of Pediatrics considers most medications to be compatible with breastfeeding.

For women with untreated or undertreated mental illness, substance use often becomes a coping mechanism. Although there is little literature on this topic, proper treatment of mental illness, which may include being stabilized on medications, can help decrease a woman's substance use during pregnancy.

Pharmacokinetics of the maternal-fetal-placental unit

The free fraction of almost all drugs has been shown to cross the placenta and enter the fetal circulation in measurable quantities. Several models have been used to explain the pharmacokinetics of the maternal-fetal-placental unit. The majority of these models suggest two main factors that contribute to pharmacokinetic changes due to pregnancy:

- maternal physiological changes, including delayed gastric emptying, decreased gastrointestinal motility, increased volume of distribution, decreased drug binding capacity, decreased levels of plasma protein (albumin), increased hepatic metabolism due to liver enzyme induction and increased renal clearance

- the effect of the placental-fetal compartment.

These factors can affect any or all of drug absorption, distribution, metabolism and elimination. Therefore, the degree and nature of the changes in the pharmacokinetic profile of a given drug due to pregnancy depend on the changes in metabolic pathways to which the agent is susceptible.

Teratogenicity and fetal toxicity

Teratogenesis is the structural or functional dysgenesis of fetal organs and/or skeletal structures. The typical manifestations include fetal growth restriction or death, carcinogenesis and physical malformations, and they may be of varying severity, requiring surgery in extreme cases.

Some drugs are not considered teratogenic but, rather, *fetotoxic*. These agents are not considered to cause physical birth defects per se but are known to have harmful health effects on the fetus and child following long-term exposure in utero.

A prime example of a substance that is both teratogenic and fetotoxic is alcohol, which can cause physical defects when used in early pregnancy and adverse long-term neurodevelopmental effects when used heavily throughout pregnancy.

Breastfeeding recommendations

Many drugs can be taken while breastfeeding without harm to the infant. The American Academy of Pediatrics considers excretion of less than 10 per cent of a drug into the breast milk to be compatible with breastfeeding.[2]

The recommendations in this handbook are based on how a substance would affect a full-term newborn healthy baby of average weight. It is unknown how even a small amount of drug excreted into the breast milk may affect a premature, low-weight baby.

Maternal and neonatal withdrawal

Prevention and treatment of withdrawal from some psychotropic medications and other substances may require both medical intervention and psychosocial supports. Medical treatment focuses on relieving withdrawal symptoms and preventing complications for the mother and her baby. Psychosocial supports focus on helping the mother overcome cravings and dysphoria. Psychosocial support, including counselling, can also facilitate a woman's entry into treatment for withdrawal and any other potential substance use issue. In other words, withdrawal can present an important opportunity for intervention, for providing information and for educating women about use of prescription medications and other substances.

Women whose withdrawal symptoms are treated inadequately or without compassion are more likely to relapse. To best support women withdrawing from substance use, issues such as housing, poverty, nutrition, prenatal care, relationships and mental health should be addressed with an individualized long-term treatment plan. Treating and dealing with the withdrawal experience in the absence of these and other issues in the woman's life will rarely lead to her long-term substance use reduction and/or recovery.

Information about withdrawal symptoms, risks and complications in the mother and withdrawal symptoms in the newborn is included in some of the individual drug sections that follow.

References

1. Finer, L.B. & Henshaw, S.K. (2006). Disparities in rates of unintended pregnancy in the United States, 1994 and 2001. *Perspectives on Sexual and Reproductive Health, 38* (2), 90–96.

2. Astrup-Jensen, A., Bates, C.J., Begg, E.J., Edwards, S., Lazarus, C., Matheson, I. et al. (1996). Use of the monographs on drugs. In P.N. Bennett (Ed.), *Drugs and Human Lactation* (pp. 67–74). Amsterdam: Elsevier.

Alcohol

Although a legal and socially accepted drug, alcohol poses a health risk to the developing fetus when consumed during pregnancy. Alcohol crosses the placenta and can reach the fetus at levels similar to those in the mother. Since alcohol is the most widely used human teratogen among women of reproductive age, alcohol consumption during pregnancy is the leading preventable cause of neurodevelopmental deficits in Canada. A safe threshold for prenatal alcohol exposure has never been determined.[1]

SUMMARY AND RECOMMENDATIONS

- The more alcohol consumed, the higher the risks of major malformations, spontaneous abortion and other effects. Consequently, heavy drinking (often defined as more than two standard drinks per day) and/or binge drinking (when a person consumes five or more standard drinks on one occasion) is considered most harmful.[2]

- Discontinuing alcohol consumption at any time during pregnancy can improve the health outcome for the fetus.[3]

- Good nutrition throughout pregnancy is recommended, which includes taking a prenatal multivitamin once per day during pregnancy.

- Breastfeeding women should plan ahead and pump their milk for later use before occasions when they expect to consume alcohol (e.g., social events).[4] (See Figure 4 on page 42.)

Fetal effects

Major malformations

Consuming alcohol while pregnant increases the risk of harm to the baby, including stillbirths, growth restrictions and facial, skeletal, kidney and cardiac defects.[5,6]

Spontaneous abortion

One study[7] reports that in over 5,000 pregnant women who consumed alcohol moderately (defined in the study as 3.5 drinks per week) the risk of first trimester spontaneous abortion increased significantly.

Neonatal effects

Newborns can experience withdrawal symptoms of varying severity when the mother is intoxicated during delivery. Common examples include tremors and ventricular tachycardia (a potentially fatal disruption of normal heartbeat). Some newborns will experience severe withdrawal symptoms, such as seizures. In one study, acute withdrawal symptoms were detected in 24 per cent of newborns whose mothers had consumed alcohol close to delivery.[7]

Long-term effects on the child

Fetal alcohol spectrum disorder

Fetal alcohol spectrum disorder (FASD) is an umbrella term that describes the range of physical and neurological effects that can occur in people exposed to alcohol during pregnancy. This disorder is found in approximately one per cent of all births and manifests as brain damage, usually in the absence of obvious physical signs.[7] The neurological effects may be in the form of abnormal cognition or social behaviour. Symptoms of FASD may have lifelong implications for an individual.[7]

Fetal alcohol syndrome

Fetal alcohol syndrome (FAS) is the most severe and clinically recognizable form of alcohol damage caused in utero. The syndrome's characteristics include a pattern of distinct facial features, prenatal and postnatal growth retardation, and functional or structural central nervous system abnormalities. FAS is caused by heavy drinking throughout pregnancy, and it is estimated that 4.3 per cent of pregnant women who drink heavily will have babies with FAS.[8] Several sources state that chronic maternal ingestion of at least 2g/kg/day of alcohol (i.e., about eight standard drinks per occasion) is associated with FAS.[9]

FAS is most easily diagnosed between the ages of eight months and eight years.[10,3] Early diagnosis and treatment (i.e., prior to six years of age) has been found to considerably improve the long-term outcome for these children.

Breastfeeding

Alcohol enters the mother's breast milk at levels similar to maternal blood levels, yet the elimination rate from the baby's body occurs at half the rate of an adult's. There are potential risks for a baby who receives alcohol. With excessive amounts of alcohol, these risks include possible impairment of the baby's motor development, changes in his or her sleep patterns and the baby's refusal to nurse due to a change in the milk's flavour. High doses of alcohol can also reduce the mother's rate of milk production.[4]

Figure 4 on the next page shows an algorithm, created by Motherisk, to calculate how long it will take for alcohol to be eliminated from a woman's breast milk.

Figure 4: Breastfeeding algorithm[4]

Time from beginning of drinking until clearance of alcohol from breast milk for women of various body weights: *Assuming alcohol metabolism is constant at 15 mg/dL and woman is of average height (1.62 m [5'4"]).*

MOTHER'S WEIGHT KG (LB)	NUMBER OF DRINKS* (HOURS : MINUTES)											
	1	2	3	4	5	6	7	8	9	10	11	12
40.8 (90)	2:50	5:40	8:30	11:20	14:10	17:00	19:51	22:41				
43.1 (95)	2:46	5:32	8:19	11:05	13:52	16:38	19:25	22:11				
45.4 (100)	2:42	5:25	8:08	10:51	13:34	16:17	19:00	21:43				
47.6 (105)	2:39	5:19	7:58	10:38	13:18	15:57	18:37	21:16	23:56			
49.9 (110)	2:36	5:12	7:49	10:25	13:01	15:38	18:14	20:50	23:27			
52.2 (115)	2:33	5:06	7:39	10:12	12:46	15:19	17:52	20:25	22:59			
54.4 (120)	2:30	5:00	7:30	10:00	12:31	15:01	17:31	20:01	22:32			
56.7 (125)	2:27	4:54	7:22	9:49	12:16	14:44	17:11	19:38	22:06			
59.0 (130)	2:24	4:49	7:13	9:38	12:03	14:27	16:52	19:16	21:41			
61.2 (135)	2:21	4:43	7:05	9:27	11:49	14:11	16:33	18:55	21:17	23:39		
63.5 (140)	2:19	4:38	6:58	9:17	11:37	13:56	16:15	18:35	20:54	23:14		
65.8 (145)	2:16	4:33	6:50	9:07	11:24	13:41	15:58	18:15	20:32	22:49		
68.0 (150)	2:14	4:29	6:43	8:58	11:12	13:27	15:41	17:56	20:10	22:25		
70.3 (155)	2:12	4:24	6:36	8:18	11:01	13:13	15:25	17:37	19:49	22:02		
72.6 (160)	2:10	4:20	6:30	8:10	10:50	13:00	15:10	17:20	19:30	21:40	23:50	
74.8 (165)	2:07	4:15	6:23	8:31	10:39	12:47	14:54	17:02	19:10	21:18	23:50	
77.1 (170)	2:06	4:11	6:17	8:23	10:28	12:34	14:40	16:46	18:51	20:57	23:03	
79.3 (175)	2:03	4:07	6:11	8:14	10:18	12:22	14:26	16:29	18:33	20:37	22:40	
81.6 (180)	2:01	4:03	6:05	8:07	10:08	12:10	14:12	16:14	18:15	20:17	22:19	
83.9 (185)	1:59	3:59	5:59	7:59	9:59	11:59	13:59	15:59	17:58	19:58	21:58	23:58
86.2 (190)	1:58	3:56	5:54	7:52	9:50	11:48	13:46	15:44	17:42	19:40	21:38	23:36
88.5 (196)	1:56	3:52	5:48	7:44	9:41	11:37	13:33	15:29	17:26	19:22	21:18	23:14
90.7 (200)	1:54	3:49	5:43	7:38	9:32	11:27	13:21	15:16	17:10	19:06	20:59	22:54
93.0 (206)	1:52	3:45	5:38	7:31	9:24	11:17	13:09	15:02	16:55	18:48	20:41	22:34
95.3 (210)	1:51	3:42	5:33	7:24	9:16	11:07	12:58	14:48	16:41	18:32	20:23	22:14

* 1 drink = 340 g (12 oz) of 5% beer or 141.75 g (5 oz) of 11% wine or 42.53 g (1.5 oz) of 46% liquor.
Example 1: For a 40.8 kg (90 lb) woman who consumed three drinks in 1 hour, it would take 8 hours, 30 minutes for there to be no alcohol in her breast milk but for a 95.3 kg (210 lb) woman drinking the same amount, it would take 5 hours, 33 minutes.
Example 2: For a 63.5 kg (140 lb) woman drinking four beers starting at 8:00 pm, it would take 9 hours, 17 minutes for there to be no alcohol in her breast milk (i.e. until 5:17 am).

Withdrawal effects on the mother

Withdrawal symptoms typically begin six to 12 hours after the person's last drink and peak in 24 to 72 hours.[11] The most reliable sign of withdrawal is tremor, which is most pronounced when the person reaches for an object. Anxiety, sweating, nausea, vomiting and headache are other common withdrawal symptoms. Many people do not recognize that they are in withdrawal and may attribute their tremors to anxiety.

The risk of withdrawal increases when a person consumes more than 40 drinks per week.[11] People who drink heavily and who consume alcohol at a predictable time every day should be carefully assessed for withdrawal symptoms: there is evidence that people who are alcohol dependent may experience subacute withdrawal,[12] which is characterized by insomnia, anxiety, fatigue and alcohol cravings, and may last for months.

Alcohol withdrawal can trigger grand mal seizures (sudden loss of consciousness together with convulsions); other complications include arrhythmia, hallucinations and delirium tremens (a dangerous syndrome consisting of hallucinations, extreme confusion, fever and tachycardia). (Note: Delirium tremens is rarely seen in younger, otherwise healthy patients.)

References

1. Koren, G., Caprara, D., Chan, D., Jacobson, S. & Porter, K. (2004). Motherisk update: Is it all right to drink a little during pregnancy? *Canadian Family Physician, 50,* 1643–1644.

2. Martinez-Frias, M.L., Bermejo, E., Rodriguez-Pinilla, E. & Frias, J.L. (2004). Risk for congenital anomalies associated with different sporadic and daily doses of alcohol consumption during pregnancy: A case-control study. *Birth Defects Research. Part A, Clinical and Molecular Teratology, 70* (4), 194–200.

3. Streissguth, A.P., Bookstein, F.L., Barr, H.M., Sampson, P.D., O'Malley, K. & Young, J.K. (2004). Risk factors for adverse life outcomes in fetal alcohol syndrome and fetal alcohol effects. *Journal of Developmental and Behavioral Pediatrics, 25* (4), 228–238.

4. Koren, G. (2002). Drinking alcohol while breastfeeding: Will it harm my baby? *Canadian Family Physician, 48* (1), 39–41. Available: www.cfpc.ca/cfp/2002/jan/vol48-jan-clinical-1.asp. Accessed July 12, 2007.

5. Sampson, P.D., Bookstein, F.L., Barr, H.M. & Streissguth, A.P. (1994). Prenatal alcohol exposure, birthweight, and measures of child size from birth to age 14 years. *American Journal of Public Health, 84* (9), 1421–1428.

6. Chudley, A.E., Conry, J., Cook, J.L., Loock, C., Rosales, T. & LeBlanc, N. (2005). Fetal alcohol spectrum disorder: Canadian guidelines for diagnosis. *Canadian Medical Association Journal, 172* (5 Suppl.), S1–S21.

7. Windham, G.C., Von Behren, J., Fenster, L., Schaefer, C. & Swan, S.H. (1997). Moderate maternal alcohol consumption and risk of spontaneous abortion. *Epidemiology, 8* (5), 509–514.

8. Abel, E.L. (1995). An update on incidence of FAS: FAS is not an equal opportunity birth defect. *Neurotoxicology and Teratology, 17* (4), 437–443.

9. Koren, G. (1994). *Maternal-Fetal Toxicology: A Clinician's Guide* (2nd ed.). New York: Marcel Dekker.

10. Romera Modamio, G., Fernández López, A., Jordán García, Y., Pastor Gómez, A., Rodriguez Miguélez, J.M., Botet Mussons, F. et al. (1997). Alcoholic embryofetopathy: Neonatal case reports for the past twelve years. *Anales Españoles de Pediatria, 47* (4), 405–409.

11. Kahan, M. & Wilson, L. (2002). *Managing Alcohol, Tobacco and Other Drug Problems: A Pocket Guide for Physicians and Nurses.* Toronto: Centre for Addiction and Mental Health.

12. Hornyak, M., Haas, P., Veit, J., Gann, H. & Riemann, D. (2004). Magnesium treatment of primary alcohol-dependent patients during subacute withdrawal: An open pilot study with polysomnography. *Alcoholism: Clinical and Experimental Research, 28* (11), 1702–1709.

Amphetamines

Examples

Amphetamine, dextroamphetamine (Dexedrine), methylphenidate (Ritalin), methamphetamine

Street names

Speed, bennies, glass, crank, pep pills, uppers, meth (also used to refer to methadone), chalk, ice, crystal, crystal meth, jib

Amphetamines are stimulant drugs used to treat such disorders as attention-deficit/hyperactivity disorder, narcolepsy and refractory depression. When amphetamines are used therapeutically, they are ingested orally. However, when they are abused, they can not only be ingested orally, but also snorted, smoked (e.g., crystal meth) or injected.

SUMMARY AND RECOMMENDATIONS

- If the benefits outweigh potential risks, therapeutic use of amphetamines at the lowest dose possible may be continued during pregnancy. However, amphetamine use during pregnancy at higher-than-recommended dosages, or abuse of amphetamines, are not recommended.

- Even if a woman is abusing amphetamines, it is important to provide her with non-judgmental support and to keep her with her baby. There is no clinical reason to keep the baby away from the mother and there are known benefits of keeping mother and child together.

- Careful monitoring of the neonates of mothers who used amphetamines while pregnant is recommended, and may need to continue longer than for babies born to mothers who used cocaine while pregnant (methamphetamine, in particular, has a long half-life). Comfort measures—especially touch, reduced stimulation (e.g., a quiet room with dim lighting) and breastfeeding—are generally sufficient to care for these babies. There is no pharmacological treatment for babies exposed to the mother's prenatal amphetamine use.

- Discuss with the mother the risks of breastfeeding while using amphetamines and the overall benefits of breastfeeding. Use of amphetamines should not necessarily be considered contraindicated during breastfeeding.

- Concerning crystal meth use, the baby's environment must be monitored to ensure the child is not exposed to a high-risk lifestyle (e.g., to the dangers of a crystal meth lab in the home).

Fetal effects

Amphetamines are known to constrict blood flow to the placenta, which reduces oxygen flow to the developing fetus. Data from human and animal studies about the effects of amphetamine exposure on the fetus are inconclusive.[1]

Studies suggest that problematic methamphetamine use by a woman during pregnancy may cause premature delivery and low-birth-weight babies; however, study confounders (e.g., multiple drug use) make forming a definite conclusion impossible. A thorough medical exam is necessary to exclude other medical conditions.

One study showed a correlation between women's methamphetamine use and low birth weight, but revealed no differences in head circumference, Apgar scores or gestational age as compared to controls.[2] Another study showed that babies born to mothers who abused methamphetamine had a significant decrease in gestational age, birth weight, length and head circumference.[3] A third study found that the methamphetamine-exposed group was 3.5 times more likely to be small for gestational age than the unexposed group.[4]

Major malformations

Amphetamines do not appear to be human teratogens, especially when used within a therapeutic context.[5–7]

Spontaneous abortion

Amphetamines may increase the risks of maternal hypertension, possibly leading to spontaneous abortion, but this has not been reported in the literature.

Neonatal effects

Neonatal withdrawal symptoms, which include shrill cries, irritability, jerking, sneezing, poor feeding, tremors and hypertonia, have been reported.[3,8] These babies may need increased medical support (e.g., repeated suctioning, oxygen, ventilation) immediately after delivery.

Long-term effects on the child

One study followed 66 infants of mothers who were addicted to amphetamines during pregnancy. These infants experienced some drowsiness in the first few months, but presented normal somatic and psychomotor development at one year of age.[9]

Breastfeeding

Amphetamines are excreted into breast milk and have been found in the urine of breastfeeding infants;[10] however, no adverse effects were observed in neonates during the first two years of observation. The American Academy of Pediatrics states that breastfeeding and amphetamine abuse are contraindicated, though this recommendation is not based on published data. Taking stimulants may cause irritability and poor sleeping patterns in the baby; however, there is no known data on this, and the percentage of the dose that enters breast milk is unknown. A recent report of prescribed methylphenidate use by the mother during breastfeeding measured the baby's dose as 0.2 per cent of the mother's dose.[11]

Withdrawal effects on the mother

Symptoms of withdrawal may include fatigue, nightmares, insomnia, increased appetite, psychomotor agitation or retardation, and dysphoric mood. Withdrawal from amphetamines is primarily a psychological process, and can be safely undertaken. Women should be provided supportive care and monitored for suicidal ideation.

Effects of untreated illness

While the effects of untreated ADHD during pregnancy specifically have not been studied, it has been shown that people with untreated ADHD are more likely to self-medicate through substance abuse.[12] Depending on the severity of the symptoms, treatment through behavioural and other non-pharmacological therapies should be considered. In the case of more severe symptoms—those that could put the mother's health and safety at risk—and concomitant anxiety and depression, the risks of controlled amphetamine use may be considered acceptable.

References

1. U.S. Department of Health and Human Services, National Toxicology Program, Center for the Evaluation of Risks to Human Reproduction. (2005). *NTP-CERHR Monograph on the Potential Human Reproductive and Developmental Effects of Amphetamines* (NIH Publication No. 05-4474). Research Triangle Park, NC: Author. Available: http://cerhr.niehs.nih.gov/chemicals/stimulants/amphetamines/AmphetamineMonograph.pdf. Accessed July 11, 2007.

2. Ramin, S.M., Little, B.B., Trimmer, K.J., Standard, D.I., Blakely, C.A. & Snell, L.M. (1992). Methamphetamine use during pregnancy in a large urban population [Abstract]. *American Journal of Obstetrics and Gynecology, 166,* 353.

3. Oro, A.S. & Dixon, S.D. (1987). Perinatal cocaine and methamphetamine exposure: Maternal and neonatal correlates. *Journal of Pediatrics, 111* (4), 571–578.

4. Smith, L.M., LaGasse, L.L., Derauf, C., Grant, P., Shah, R., Arria, A. et al. (2006). The infant development, environment, and lifestyle study: Effects of prenatal methamphetamine exposure, polydrug exposure, and poverty on intrauterine growth. *Pediatrics, 118* (3), 1149–1156.

5. Chernoff, G.F. & Jones, K.L. (1981). Fetal preventive medicine: Teratogens and the unborn baby. *Pediatric Annals, 10* (6), 210–217.

6. Kalter, H. & Warkany, J. (1983). Congenital malformations (second of two parts). *New England Journal of Medicine, 308* (9), 491–497.

7. Zierler, S. (1985). Maternal drugs and congenital heart disease. *Obstetrics and Gynecology, 65* (2), 155–165.

8. Sussman, S. (1963). Narcotic and methamphetamine use during pregnancy: Effect on newborn infants. *American Journal of Diseases of Children, 106,* 325–330.

9. Billing, L., Eriksson, M., Larsson, G.E. & Zetterström, R. (1980). Amphetamine addiction and pregnancy III: One year follow-up of the children—Psychosocial and pediatric aspects. *Acta Paediatrica Scandinavica, 69* (5), 675–680.

10. Steiner, E., Villén, T., Hallberg, M. & Rane, A. (1984). Amphetamine secretion in breast milk. *European Journal of Clinical Pharmacology, 27* (1), 123–124.

11. Hackett, L.P., Kristensen, J.H., Hale, T.W., Paterson, R. & Ilett, K.F. (2006). Methylphenidate and breast-feeding. *Annals of Pharmacotherapy, 40* (10), 1890–1891.

12. Kalbag, A.S. & Levin, F.R. (2005). Adult ADHD and substance abuse: Diagnostic and treatment issues. *Substance Use & Misuse, 40* (13 & 14), 1955–1981.

Antidepressants

Examples

- Selective serotonin reuptake inhibitors or SSRIs: fluoxetine (Prozac), paroxetine (Paxil), sertraline (Zoloft), citalopram (Celexa)
- Serotonin/norepinephrine reuptake inhibitors or SNRIs: venlafaxine (Effexor)
- Tricyclic antidepressants or TCAs: amitriptyline (Elavil), clomipramine (Anafranil), imipramine (Tofranil)
- Others: bupropion (Wellbutrin/Zyban), trazodone (Desyrel), mirtazapine (Remeron)

Twice as many women as men experience depression and up to 20 per cent of women of childbearing age (i.e., ages 14 to 46) are diagnosed with the condition.[1] Depression is most prevalent between ages 25 and 44 for both women and men: approximately 10 to 15 per cent of these women experience depression during pregnancy and postpartum. Antidepressants are used to treat several anxiety disorders and are prescribed for these disorders in rates similar to those for depression. A substantial proportion of women are therefore likely to be taking antidepressants when they become pregnant.

SUMMARY AND RECOMMENDATIONS

Current evidence suggests that, as a group, antidepressants are relatively safe to take during pregnancy and breastfeeding and that women should not abruptly discontinue their use.

- In cases where women are taking antidepressants during late pregnancy, babies should be observed for longer than one to two days postpartum to detect possible neonatal symptomatology (e.g., respiratory distress, constant crying, convulsions).
- Since babies may react differently to even very small amounts of a drug, if a mother is taking antidepressants while breastfeeding, her baby should be observed for any changes (e.g., drowsiness, difficulty feeding).
- Women should be reassured about the safety of antidepressant use. Emerging evidence strongly suggests that untreated depression poses its own risk, not only to maternal health but also to the infant's health.[2] A woman who is in optimal mental health is equipped to give the best possible care to her baby.

Fetal effects

Major malformations

Tricyclic antidepressants have been on the market since 1958 and, as a group, they are not associated with an increased risk for major malformations.[3] The newer antidepressants have also not been found to increase this risk.[4,5]

In fall 2005, GlaxoSmithKline published on its website the results of a claims database study, which found that infants exposed to paroxetine may be at higher risk of congenital malformations, in particular cardiovascular defects. The study was based on outcomes of 815 infants; the reported incidence of cardiovascular malformations, unspecified in terms of severity, was two per cent.[6] An update was presented at a meeting in 2006, in which the data had been re-analyzed and the incidence was adjusted to 1.5 per cent.[7]

A recent study[8] reported the outcomes of 1,170 cases, collected prospectively from teratogen information services throughout the world, of infants who were exposed to paroxetine in the first trimester of pregnancy. These infants were compared to a non-exposed cohort to determine the rates of cardiovascular defects. The rate of heart defects in the paroxetine group was 0.8 per cent versus 0.7 per cent in the non-exposed group, both of which are within the range of expected cardiovascular malformations in the general population.

In 2006, a study documented a one per cent increased risk for persistent pulmonary hypertension in the newborns of mothers who took SSRIs during pregnancy.[9]

Spontaneous abortion

Several studies that examined antidepressant use during pregnancy have suggested an increased rate of spontaneous abortions in women exposed to antidepressants compared to non-exposed women; however, the results were not statistically significant due to the small sample sizes. A meta-analysis of these studies, conducted to determine baseline rates for spontaneous abortions and antidepressant effects, found that the rate of spontaneous abortions was significantly higher (i.e., by 3.9 per cent) in women taking antidepressants. The class of antidepressants taken did not affect the rate.[10] (This increase may be related to depression itself, rather than to the effects of antidepressants.)

Neonatal effects

Poor neonatal adaptation has been reported in some babies following in utero exposure to antidepressants, with increased admissions to neonatal intensive care units.[11] Clinical manifestation of poor neonatal adaptation includes such usually transient and self-limiting symptoms as jitteriness, tachycardia, hypothermia, vomiting, hypoglycemia, irritability, constant crying, increased tonus, eating and sleeping difficulties, convulsions and respiratory distress. This pattern of symptoms may occur in up to 30 per cent of all babies exposed to SSRIs during late pregnancy. However, in studies with comparative groups, this same pattern of symptoms occurred in six to nine per cent of babies who were not exposed to antidepressants in late pregnancy.[11]

Long-term effects on the child

To determine whether fluoxetine and TCAs cause adverse neurodevelopmental sequelae, researchers conducted a long-term assessment of children's temperament, mood, arousability, activity level, distractibility and, most importantly, global IQ and language development.[12] The assessment found no association between gestational use of TCAs or fluoxetine and any of the outcomes that were examined.

By contrast, for women with untreated depression, the child's global IQ and language development showed negative effects in relation to the duration of the depression and the number of postnatal depressive episodes. These results suggest that children of mothers with depression have decreased global IQ and language development as compared to children of non-depressed women.[12] Another study found similar results: in a case where internalizing behaviours (e.g., depression, anxiety and withdrawal) were examined in four-year-old children of mothers who had taken SSRIs while pregnant, the mother's impaired mood had an identified impact on her child.[13]

Breastfeeding

Most antidepressants are excreted into breast milk in small amounts and, as a group, are considered compatible with breastfeeding.[14] Of the SSRIs, fluoxetine is excreted in the highest amount (i.e., five to nine per cent of the maternal dose enters the breast milk.)

Despite the relative safety of using antidepressants while breastfeeding, providers should be aware that babies may react differently even to very small amounts of the drug. It is important to observe babies for changes such as drowsiness and difficulty feeding.

Withdrawal effects on the mother

Many women who are pregnant or breastfeeding abruptly discontinue taking their antidepressant medication,[15] but such sudden cessation may cause the mother to experience discontinuation symptoms or re-emergence of the depression. The discontinuation symptoms, which tend to occur within days of stopping treatment, may include general somatic, gastrointestinal, and affective and sleep disturbances. Recurrence of the depression occurs gradually, and usually within weeks. While reinstituting the antidepressant medication mitigates the discontinuation symptoms (within 24 hours), the depression may take several weeks to respond to treatment.

One study reported that 11 out of 36 women who abruptly discontinued their antidepressant reported suicidal ideation; four were admitted to hospital.[15]

Effects of untreated illness

Untreated depression during pregnancy appears to carry substantial risks to the mother, fetus and infant, including risks due to unhealthy maternal behaviours arising from the depression (e.g., suicidal ideation) and an increased risk for spontaneous abortion, hypertension, pre-eclampsia, lower birth weight and postpartum depression.

A 2006 study of pregnant women diagnosed with depression who were followed longitudinally throughout their pregnancies found that pregnancy does not have a protective effect against depression and concluded that women should be treated with antidepressants if necessary.[16] Depression in the mother can impact a child's emotional and cognitive development;[2] a depressed or withdrawn mother may fail to bond with her baby or respond to her infant's cues (e.g., cooing in response to her baby, making eye contact).

Taken as a whole, the evidence suggests that untreated depression, rather than treatment with antidepressants during pregnancy, results in adverse outcomes.[2]

References

1. Bhatia, S.C. & Bhatia, S.K. (1999). Depression in women: Diagnostic and treatment considerations. *American Family Physician, 60* (1), 225–234, 239–240.

2. Bonari, L., Pinto, N., Ahn, E., Einarson, A., Steiner, M. & Koren, G. (2004). Perinatal risks of untreated depression during pregnancy. *Canadian Journal of Psychiatry, 49* (11), 726–735.

3. Altshuler, L.L., Cohen, L., Szuba, M.P., Burt, V.K., Gitlin, M. & Mintz, J. (1996). Pharmacologic management of psychiatric illness during pregnancy: Dilemmas and guidelines. *American Journal of Psychiatry, 153* (5), 592–606.

4. Einarson, T.R. & Einarson, A. (2005). Newer antidepressants in pregnancy and rates of major malformations: A meta-analysis of prospective comparative studies. *Pharmacoepidemiology and Drug Safety, 14* (12), 823–827.

5. Djulus, J., Koren, G., Einarson, T.R., Wilton, L., Shakir, S., Diav-Citrin, O. et al. (2006). Exposure to mirtazapine during pregnancy: A prospective, comparative study of birth outcomes. *Journal of Clinical Psychiatry, 67* (8), 1280–1284.

6. GlaxoSmithKline Advisory. October 2005. Available: http://ctr.gsk.co.uk/welcome.asp. Accessed October 27, 2006.

7. Cole, A., Ng, E., Ephross, S., Cosmatos, I. & Walker, A. (2006, August). *Paroxetine in the First Trimester and Prevalence of Congenital Malformations.* Abstract presented at the 22nd International Conference on Pharmacoepidemiology and Therapeutic Risk Management.

8. Einarson, A., Pistelli, A., DeSantis, M., Chambers, C.D., Malm, H., Paulus, W.E. et al. (2007, June). *Paroxetine Use in Pregnancy: Is There an Association with Congenital Cardiovascular Defects?* Abstract presented at the meeting of the Teratology Society, Pittsburgh, PA.

9. Chambers, C.D., Hernandez-Diaz, S., Van Marter, L.J., Werler, M.M., Louik, C., Jones, K.L. et al. (2006). Selective serotonin-reuptake inhibitors and risk of persistent pulmonary hypertension of the newborn. *New England Journal of Medicine, 354* (6), 579–587.

10. Hemels, M.E., Einarson, A., Koren, G., Lanctôt, K.L. & Einarson, T.R. (2005). Antidepressant use during pregnancy and the rates of spontaneous abortions: A meta-analysis. *Annals of Pharmacotherapy, 39* (5), 803–809.

11. Koren, G., Matsui, D., Einarson, A., Knoppert, D. & Steiner, M. (2005). Is maternal use of selective serotonin reuptake inhibitors in the third trimester of pregnancy harmful to neonates? *Canadian Medical Association Journal, 172* (11), 1457–1459.

12. Nulman, I., Rovet, J., Stewart, D.E., Wolpin, J., Gardner, H.A., Theis, J.G. et al. (1997). Neurodevelopment of children exposed in utero to antidepressant drugs. *New England Journal of Medicine, 336* (4), 258–262.

13. Misri, S., Reebye, P., Kendrick, K., Carter, D., Ryan, D., Grunau, R.E. et al. (2006). Internalizing behaviors in 4-year-old children exposed in utero to psychotropic medications. *American Journal of Psychiatry, 163* (6), 1026–1032.

14. Hale, T.W. (2006). *Medications and Mothers' Milk: A Manual of Lactational Pharmacology* (12th ed.) (pp. 113, 365, 613, 814–815, 871, 895). Amarillo, TX: Hale Publishing.

15. Einarson, A., Selby, P. & Koren, G. (2001). Abrupt discontinuation of psychotropic drugs during pregnancy: Fear of teratogenic risk and impact of counselling. *Journal of Psychiatry and Neuroscience, 26* (1), 44–48.

16. Cohen, L.S., Altshuler, L.L., Harlow, B.L., Nonacs, R., Newport, D.J., Viguera, A.C. et al. (2006). Relapse of major depression during pregnancy in women who maintain or discontinue antidepressant treatment. *Journal of the American Medical Association, 295* (5), 499–507.

Antiepileptics

Examples

Older antiepileptics: carbamazepine (Tegretol), phenytoin (Dilantin), divalproex/valproate/valproic acid (Epival)

Newer antiepileptics: lamotrigine (Lamictal), gabapentin (Neurontin), oxcarbazepine (Trileptal), topiramate (Topamax)

Antiepileptics are frequently used to treat bipolar disorder, in addition to epilepsy.

Epilepsy is one the most commonly encountered neurological disorders in obstetrics. Incidence of seizure disorder during pregnancy is estimated at 0.3 to 0.5 per cent.[1] Compared to the general obstetric population, having epilepsy while pregnant is considered high risk, mainly due to the teratogenic potential of antiepileptic drugs and increased risk of maternal, fetal and neonatal complications (e.g., hypertension, pre-eclampsia, antepartum hemorrhage, caesarean delivery, stillbirth, neonatal death, intrauterine growth retardation, preterm delivery).

SUMMARY AND RECOMMENDATIONS

- Careful clinical management is extremely important because bipolar symptoms and/or seizure frequency can change during pregnancy, and both seizure activity and antiepileptic drug treatment can affect the developing fetus. Women should be treated with the drug that controls their disorder and, if at all possible, with monotherapy at the lowest effective dose.

- Antiepileptics should never be abruptly discontinued because of the consequences to both the mother and the fetus.

- Folic acid (four milligrams per day) should be taken for three months prior to conception and during the first trimester to help prevent folic acid deficiency–induced malformations (i.e., neural tube defects).

- Women should be offered a detailed ultrasound examination and their levels of maternal serum alpha-fetoproteins should be monitored.

- With proper prenatal and postpartum management, up to 95 per cent of pregnancies in which women took antiepileptics are reported to have had favourable outcomes.[2]

Fetal effects

Major malformations

OLDER ANTIEPILEPTICS

Use of older antiepileptics during pregnancy increases the risk of major malformations:

- Phenytoin increases the risk of neural tube defects by approximately 10 per cent (highest overall rate).[3]

- Valproic acid increases the risk of neural tube defects by approximately five to nine per cent.[3]

- Carbamazepine increases the risk of neural tube defects by approximately one per cent (lowest teratogenic effect).[3]

NEWER ANTIEPILEPTICS

Use of some newer antiepileptics during pregnancy minimally increases the rate of neural tube defects:

- Lamotrigine: Preliminary data from pregnancy registries around the world suggest no increased risk for birth defects with the use of lamotrigine.[4] However, the North American Antiepileptic Drug Pregnancy Registry suggests a potential increased risk for non-syndromic cleft palate, which was observed among 564 exposed infants: three infants had isolated cleft palate, two had isolated cleft lip. This prevalence of oral clefts (0.89 per cent) is higher than the 0.037 per cent observed in the control group.[5]

- Gabapentin: The Gabapentin Pregnancy Registry assessed the safety of gabapentin exposure during pregnancy in 39 cases and found no increased risk for major malformations.[6]

- Topiramate: Only a few case reports exist of infants exposed to topiramate in utero, with no major malformations cited.[1]

- Oxcarbazepine: A study of 309 pregnancies, 248 with maternal exposure to monotherapy and 61 with exposure to adjunctive therapy, cited six malformations among infants of mothers in the monotherapy group. This malformation rate of 2.4 per cent in the monotherapy group is within the baseline range for the general population.[7]

Spontaneous abortion

A 1988 study found no increase in spontaneous abortion in pregnant women taking antiepileptic medications.[8] There is no data available on the risk of spontaneous abortion with newer antiepileptics.

Neonatal effects

There are no reports of adverse neonatal effects resulting from a woman taking either older or newer antiepileptics.

Long-term effects on the child

One study[9] followed 36 pregnant women exposed to either carbamazepine or phenytoin monotherapy. Children exposed in utero to carbamazepine did not differ from children in the control groups in any of the administered neurobehavioural tests with respect to global IQ. However, on average, children in the phenytoin group scored 10 points lower on a measure of global IQ, and significantly more children in the phenytoin group had IQ scores of less than 84.8.

Another study[10] examined children exposed in utero to various antiepileptic drugs (monotherapy and polytherapy) into adolescence. This study found that maternal epilepsy and antiepileptic drug therapy during pregnancy appears to have long-term effects well into adolescence. These effects manifest in abnormal EEG patterns, minor neurologic dysfunction and poorer intellectual performance. The polytherapy group showed the most marked severity of effects. A recent review of studies examining possible neurobehavioural effects of valproic acid all reported that despite the different study designs and varied outcomes and cognitive tests, developmental delays and cognitive deficits were associated with valproic acid use in pregnancy—with the most prominent effect being on verbal IQ.[11]

Breastfeeding

Less than five per cent of the mother's dose of any antiepileptic drug is excreted into breast milk. Antiepileptics can therefore be used safely during breastfeeding.[12]

Withdrawal effects on the mother

One individual who took carbamazepine for trigeminal neuralgia became psychotic following abrupt discontinuation of the drug.[13] Three cases of acute withdrawal symptoms following gabapentin withdrawal have been documented.[14] In another report, 10 patients who abruptly stopped taking carbamazepine or phenytoin had changes in cardiac rhythm; three patients had a 10-fold increase in the rate of ventricular premature beats.[15]

Effects of untreated illness

Pregnancy does not protect against mood fluctuations in women with untreated bipolar disorder. Maintenance of euthymia during pregnancy is critical because relapse during this period strongly predicts a difficult postpartum course.

It is suspected, though not proven, that women with untreated epilepsy have a higher than baseline risk for giving birth to a child with malformations. Epilepsy per se has been thought to represent a teratogenic risk. A meta-analysis, however, found that the risk for congenital malformations in the children of mothers with untreated epilepsy was no higher than among the control group of women without epilepsy.[2]

References

1. Yerby, M.S. (2003). Clinical care of pregnant women with epilepsy: Neural tube defects and folic acid supplementation. *Epilepsia, 44* (Suppl. 3), 33–40.

2. Fried, S., Kozer, E., Nulman, I., Einarson, T.R. & Koren, G. (2004). Malformation rates in children of women with untreated epilepsy: A meta-analysis. *Drug Safety: An International Journal of Medical Toxicology and Drug Experience, 27* (3), 197–202.

3. Wyszynski, D.F., Nambisan, M., Surve, T., Alsdorf, R.M., Smith, C.R. & Holmes, L.B. (2005). Increased rate of major malformations in offspring exposed to valproate during pregnancy. *Neurology, 64* (6), 961–965.

4. Cunnington, M. & Tennis, P. (2005). Lamotrigine and the risk of malformations in pregnancy. *Neurology, 64* (6), 955–960.

5. Holmes, L.B. (2006). Increased risk for non-syndromic cleft palate among infants exposed to lamotrigine during pregnancy [Abstract]. *Teratology, 76* (5), 318.

6. Montouris, G. (2003). Gabapentin exposure in human pregnancy: Results from the Gabapentin Pregnancy Registry. *Epilepsy & Behavior, 4* (3), 310–317.

7. Montouris, G. (2005). Safety of the newer antiepileptic drug oxcarbazepine during pregnancy. *Current Medical Research and Opinion, 21* (5), 693–701.

8. Annegers, J.F., Baumgartner, K.B., Hauser, W.A. & Kurland, W.T. (1988). Epilepsy, antiepileptic drugs, and the risk of spontaneous abortion. *Epilepsia, 29* (4), 451–458.

9. Scolnik, D., Nulman, I., Rovet, J., Gladstone, D., Czchta, D., Gardner, H.A. et al (1994). Neurodevelopment of children exposed in utero to phenytoin and carbamazepine monotherapy. *Journal of the American Medical Association, 271* (10), 767–770.

10. Dean, J.C., Hailey, H., Moore, S.J., Lloyd, D.J., Turnpenny, P.D. & Little, J. (2002). Long term health and neurodevelopment in children exposed to antiepileptic drugs before birth. *Journal of Medical Genetics, 39* (4), 251–259.

11. Koren, G., Nava-Ocampo, A.A., Moretti, M.E., Sussman, R. & Nulman, I. (2006). Major malformations with valproic acid [Review]. *Canadian Family Physician, 52* (4), 441–447.

12. Crawford, P. (2005). Best practice guidelines for the management of women with epilepsy. *Epilepsia, 46* (Suppl. 9), 117–124.

13. Heh, C.W., Sramek, J., Herrera, J. & Costa, J. (1988). Exacerbation of psychosis after discontinuation of carbamazepine treatment. *American Journal of Psychiatry, 145* (7), 878–879.

14. Pittenger, C. & Desan, P.H. (2007). Gabapentin abuse, and delirium tremens upon gabapentin withdrawal. *Journal of Clinical Psychiatry, 68* (3), 483–484.

15. Kenneback, G., Ericson, M., Tomson, T. & Bergfeldt, L. (1997). Changes in arrhythmia profile and heart rate variability during abrupt withdrawal of antiepileptic drugs: Implications for sudden death. *Seizure: The Journal of the British Epilepsy Association, 6* (5), 369–375.

Antipsychotics

Examples

Typical antipsychotics: chlorpromazine (Largactil), haloperidol (Haldol), loxapine (Loxapac), perphenazine (Trilafon)

Atypical antipsychotics: clozapine (Clozaril), olanzapine (Zyprexa), quetiapine (Seroquel), risperidone (Risperdal)

Approximately one to two per cent of the population, many of them women of childbearing age, live with schizophrenia,[1] for which the older typical and newer atypical antipsychotics are prescribed. Atypicals are also prescribed for other psychiatric conditions (e.g., bipolar disorder, postpartum psychotic depression).

SUMMARY AND RECOMMENDATIONS

- A woman who requires antipsychotic medication during pregnancy and in the postpartum period should not change her treatment, if the medication is controlling her illness well. Treatment helps her to function well and be better equipped to adequately interact with and care for her baby.

TYPICAL ANTIPSYCHOTICS

- Infants exposed to typical antipsychotics in the latter part of pregnancy should be watched carefully after birth for extrapyramidal symptoms such as severe rigidity and muscle spasms.

- Infants whose mothers are taking typical antipsychotics while breastfeeding should be monitored carefully for signs of drowsiness or lethargy.

ATYPICAL ANTIPSYCHOTICS

- Although there are no documented reports of adverse effects in neonates of mothers who took atypical antipsychotics during pregnancy, these babies should be monitored for several days following their birth for possible extrapyramidal symptoms.

- Infants of mothers taking atypical antipsychotics while breastfeeding should be monitored carefully for signs of drowsiness or lethargy.

- Due to the increased risk of diabetes associated with taking atypical antipsychotics, a woman's blood sugar levels should also be monitored.

Fetal effects

TYPICAL ANTIPSYCHOTICS

The Collaborative Perinatal Project, conducted in Boston in the 1970s, monitored 142 mother-child pairs exposed to chlorpromazine during the first trimester. The project found that perinatal mortality rates and birth weights were similar to those for the general population.[2]

ATYPICAL ANTIPSYCHOTICS

Little information is available on the safety of atypical antipsychotics. A single study, documenting 151 pregnancy outcomes in exposed women, found a higher rate of low birth weight (i.e., 10 per cent in exposed babies versus two per cent in the comparison group).[3]

Major malformations

TYPICAL ANTIPSYCHOTICS

Chlorpromazine exposure has not been found to increase risk for major malformations.[2] In a study that assessed the safety of haloperidol and penfluridol in 215 pregnancies, rates of major malformations did not differ between the antipsychotic-exposed group and the control group.[4]

ATYPICAL ANTIPSYCHOTICS

In the single study available, no pregnancy outcomes showed any statistically significant differences of interest.[3]

Spontaneous abortion

TYPICAL ANTIPSYCHOTICS

Data on typical antipsychotic use and spontaneous abortion are not available.

ATYPICAL ANTIPSYCHOTICS

One study[3] documents a higher spontaneous abortion rate in the group of women taking atypical antipsychotics (22 [or 14.5 per cent]) than in the group of women not taking atypical antipsychotics (13 [or 8.6 per cent]).

Neonatal effects

TYPICAL ANTIPSYCHOTICS

In a number of babies exposed in utero to typical antipsychotics, extrapyramidal symptoms (e.g., severe rigidity, muscle spasms, shaking or restlessness) caused by the mother's use of antipsychotics while pregnant have been observed, which in some cases persisted for several months. A few cases of paralytic ileus have also been reported; however, most reports describing typical antipsychotic use in pregnancy conclude that there are no adverse effects on the neonate.[5]

ATYPICAL ANTIPSYCHOTICS

There are no reports of adverse neonatal effects in newborns exposed in utero to atypical antipsychotics.

Long-term effects on the child

TYPICAL ANTIPSYCHOTICS

Intelligence quotients of 1,309 four-year-olds born to women taking typical antipsychotic drugs during the first four lunar months of their pregnancy were similar to those of 48,973 four-year-old children of non-exposed women.[2]

ATYPICAL ANTIPSYCHOTICS

There are no studies on possible long-term effects of a mother's atypical antipsychotic use.

Breastfeeding

TYPICAL ANTIPSYCHOTICS

Less than three per cent of the maternal dose of typical antipsychotics is excreted into the breast milk. Reports of drowsiness and lethargy in some infants have been documented, although many studies cite no adverse effects.[6]

ATYPICAL ANTIPSYCHOTICS

Less than five per cent of quetiapine is excreted into the breast milk;[7] no reports of adverse effects of any other atypical antipsychotics on breastfeeding infants have been cited.

Withdrawal effects on the mother

Abrupt discontinuation of antipsychotic drugs, or a change from typical to atypical agents, can cause severe withdrawal and result in adverse physical symptoms, including exacerbation of the psychosis.[8]

Effects of untreated illness

Reports of adverse effects of untreated psychotic illness have been documented (e.g., polyserositis, rebound phenomenon, rapid relapse).[9]

In women who are pregnant or breastfeeding, untreated schizophrenia has been linked with higher rates of smoking, maternal malnutrition, low socioeconomic status, refusal or inability to take part in prenatal care, worsening of psychotic symptoms during pregnancy, poorer interaction between mother and baby, and increased suicide risk.[10]

Babies born to mothers with schizophrenia have a small but statistically significant increased risk of small size for gestational age, preterm delivery and low birth weight.[11] One study found that the risk of small size for gestational age, stillbirth, preterm delivery, low birth weight and infant death was doubled for mothers who had an acute episode during pregnancy, even controlling for higher rates of smoking in women with schizophrenia.[12] There is also an increased risk of placental abruption, infants in the lowest weight and growth decile, and congenital cardiovascular anomalies in infants born to mothers with schizophrenia.[13]

References

Morrato, E.H., Dodd, S., Oderda, G., Haxby, D.G., Allen, R. & Valuck, R.J. (2007). Prevalence, utilization patterns, and predictors of antipsychotic polypharmacy: Experience in a multistate Medicaid population, 1998–2003. *Clinical Therapeutics, 29* (1), 183–195.

Slone, D., Siskind, V., Heinonen, O.P., Monson, R.R., Kaufman, D.W. & Shapiro, S. (1977). Antenatal exposure to the phenothiazines in relation to congenital malformations, perinatal mortality rate, birth weight and intelligence quotient score. *American Journal of Obstetrics and Gynecology, 128* (5), 486–488.

McKenna, K., Koren, G., Tetelbaum, M., Wilton, L., Shakir, S., Diav-Citrin, O. et al. (2005). Pregnancy outcome of women using atypical antipsychotic drugs: A prospective comparative study. *Journal of Clinical Psychiatry, 66* (4), 444–449; Quiz 546.

Diav-Citrin, O., Shechtman, S., Ornoy, S., Arnon, J., Schaefer, C., Garbis, H. et al. (2005). Safety of haloperidol and penfluridol in pregnancy: A multicenter, prospective, controlled study. *Journal of Clinical Psychiatry, 66* (3), 317–322.

O'Connor, M., Johnson, G.H. & James, D.I. (1981). Intrauterine effects of phenothiazines. *Medical Journal of Australia, 1* (8), 416–417.

Yoshida, K., Smith, B., Craggs, M. & Kumar, R. (1998). Neuroleptic drugs in breast-milk: A study of pharmacokinetics and of possible adverse effects in breast-fed infants. *Psychological Medicine, 28* (1), 81–91.

Lee, A., Giesbrecht, E., Dunn, E. & Ito, S. (2004). Excretion of quetiapine in breast milk. *American Journal of Psychiatry, 161* (9), 1715–1716.

8. Kinon, B.J., Basson, B.R., Gilmore, J.A., Malcolm, S. & Stauffer, V.L. (2000). Strategies for switching from conventional antipsychotic drugs or risperidone to olanzapine. *Journal of Clinical Psychiatry, 61* (11), 833–840.

9. Viguera, A.C., Baldessarini, R.J., Hegarty, J.D., van Kammen, D.P. & Tohen, M. (1997). Clinical risk following abrupt and gradual withdrawal of maintenance neuroleptic treatment. *Archives of General Psychiatry, 54* (1), 49–55.

10. Usher, K., Foster, K. & McNamara, P. (2005). Antipsychotic drugs and pregnant or breastfeeding women: The issues for mental health nurses. *Journal of Psychiatric and Mental Health Nursing, 12* (6), 713–718.

11. Sacker, A., Done, D.J. & Crow, T.J. (1996). Obstetrics complications in children born of parents with schizophrenia: A meta-analysis of case-control studies. *Psychological Medicine, 26* (2), 279–287.

12. Nilsson, E., Lichtenstein, P., Cnattingius, S., Murray, R.M. & Hultman, C.M. (2002). Women with schizophrenia: Pregnancy outcome and infant death among their offspring. *Schizophrenia Research, 58* (2–3), 221–229.

13. Jablensky, A.V., Morgan, V., Zubrick, S.R., Bower, C., and Yellachich, L. (2005). Pregnancy, delivery, and neonatal complications in a population cohort of women with schizophrenia and major affective disorders. *American Journal of Psychiatry 162* (1), 79–91.

Anxiolytics/sedatives (non-benzodiazepines)

Examples

Buspirone (BuSpar); zopiclone (Imovane)

Buspirone is a psychotropic drug with anxiolytic properties, chemically unrelated to any other anti-anxiety drug, and is used to treat anxiety disorders. Zopiclone is used as an alternative treatment to benzodiazepines for the symptomatic relief of transient and short-term insomnia. Zopiclone is structurally unrelated but pharmacologically similar to benzodiazepines.

SUMMARY AND RECOMMENDATIONS

- Due to the lack of information about the use of buspirone in pregnancy and breastfeeding, it is not recommended as a drug of choice. However, if a woman is taking it and becomes pregnant, the provider should not be unduly concerned because there has been no evidence, in either animal studies or case reports, that this drug increases risk for adverse outcomes.

- While insufficient data is available to fully assess the safety of zopiclone during pregnancy, short-term use for treatment of insomnia does not appear to present undue risk.

- Zopiclone is considered safe for use during breastfeeding.

Fetal effects

Major malformations

Seventeen case reports show no evidence of buspirone increasing risk for major malformations.[1,2] One observational cohort study suggests that zopiclone does not appear to be a major human teratogen.[3] However, sufficient data is not available on either of these medications to firmly establish whether they affect the fetus during pregnancy.

Spontaneous abortion

There are no studies on whether either buspirone or zopiclone increases the risk for spontaneous abortion.

Neonatal effects

While there are reports that certain benzodiazepines taken during the last weeks of pregnancy have resulted in neonatal central nervous system depression,[5] whether or not buspirone or zopiclone could cause similar effects remains unknown. There are no case reports of adverse effects in neonates associated with the use of these non-benzodiazepine anxiolytic drugs during pregnancy.

The results of a 1999 prospective observational study on zopiclone showed no differences between the study and control groups in pregnancy outcome, fetal distress, presence of meconium at birth, preterm deliveries or neonatal intensive care admissions.[3]

Long-term effects on the child

There are no long-term studies available on the effects on the child of buspirone or zopiclone exposure in utero.

Breastfeeding

Buspirone and its metabolites are excreted into milk in rats, but no data exists on whether buspirone is excreted into human breast milk.[6] The average infant dose of zopiclone ingested through breast milk has been calculated at 1.4 per cent of the maternal dose.[7] Zopiclone is therefore considered compatible with breastfeeding.

Withdrawal effects on the mother

While withdrawal effects have not been reported with buspirone, there is a risk that anxiety symptoms may recur after abrupt discontinuation.

Withdrawal symptoms have been reported in individuals who used therapeutic or high doses of zopiclone over more than a two-week period and then abruptly discontinued use.[4] Withdrawal symptoms include rebound insomnia and anxiety, mild dysphoria and, rarely, a major withdrawal syndrome, including abdominal and muscle cramps, vomiting, sweating, tremor and convulsions.

Effects of untreated illness

There are no definitive studies on the effect of untreated anxiety or insomnia in pregnancy or postpartum.

During all three trimesters of pregnancy it is normal for women to experience changes in sleep for a variety of reasons, including high hormone levels and physical changes. The greatest sleep disturbance is typically in the first month postpartum. This may increase the risk of postpartum depression and psychosis, though this hypothesis has not been studied extensively.[8]

References

1. Wilton, L.V., Pearce, G.L., Martin, R.M., Mackay, F.J. & Mann, R.D. (1998). The outcomes of pregnancy in women exposed to newly marketed drugs in general practice in England. *British Journal of Obstetrics and Gynaecology, 105* (8), 882–889.

2. McElhatton, P.R., Garbis, H.M., Elefant, E., Vial, T., Bellemin, B., Mastroiacovo, P. et al. (1996). The outcome of pregnancy in 689 women exposed to therapeutic doses of antidepressants. A collaborative study of the European Network of Teratology Information Services (ENTIS). *Reproductive Toxicology, 10* (4), 285–294.

3. Diav-Citrin, O., Okotore, B., Lucarelli, K. & Koren, G. (1999). Pregnancy outcome following first-trimester exposure to zopiclone: A prospective controlled cohort study. *American Journal of Perinatology, 16* (4), 157–160.

4. Sanofi-Aventis Canada. (2006). *Imovane (zopiclone): Product monograph.* Laval, QU: Author.

5. McElhatton, P.R. (1994). The effects of benzodiazepine use during pregnancy and lactation. *Reproductive Toxicology, 8* (6), 461–475.

6. Bristol-Myers Squibb Canada. (2004). *BuSpar (buspirone): Product monograph.* Montreal: Author.

7. Hale, T.W. (2006). *Medications and Mothers' Milk: A Manual of Lactational Pharmacology* (12th ed.). Amarillo, TX: Hale Publishing.

8. Pien, G.W. & Schwab, R.J. (2004). Sleep disorders during pregnancy. *Sleep, 27* (7), 1405–1417.

Benzodiazepines

Examples

Alprazolam (Xanax), bromazepam (Lectopam), chlordiazepoxide (Librium), clonazepam (Rivotril), diazepam (Valium), flunitrazepam (Rohypnol), flurazepam (Dalmane), lorazepam (Ativan), midazolam (Versed), nitrazepam (Mogadon), oxazepam (Serax), temazepam (Restoril), triazolam (Halcion)

Street names

Benzos, tranks, downers

Benzodiazepines are frequently used to treat anxiety disorders,* which affect approximately 1.9 million people in Canada each year.[1] These disorders occur in women significantly more often than in men;[1] consequently, many women of childbearing age may be taking a benzodiazepine when they become pregnant.

These drugs have anticonvulsant, anxiolytic, hypnotic and sedative properties. They are used to manage anxiety disorders (including panic disorder), insomnia, seizure disorders, skeletal muscle spasticity and alcohol withdrawal, and as premedicants prior to surgical or diagnostic procedures. Benzodiazepines have also been used to manage nausea and vomiting associated with emetogenic cancer chemotherapy.

*SSRIs and SNRIs, not benzodiazepines, are generally the preferred first-line treatment for long-standing anxiety disorders.

SUMMARY AND RECOMMENDATIONS

- A woman who requires benzodiazepines during pregnancy or who has taken them prior to becoming pregnant should be advised of the conflicting information (see below), and helped to weigh the benefits of such treatment against the risks.

- A level II ultrasound can be performed to rule out visible forms of oral clefts.

- To minimize discontinuation effects on the neonate, the dose can be decreased during late pregnancy.

- During breastfeeding, the infant should be monitored for any adverse effects (e.g., drowsiness, difficulty feeding).

Fetal effects

Major malformations

Overall, there is insufficient evidence that benzodiazepines are human teratogens.[2-6] A meta-analysis of 23 studies[5] addressed the risk for congenital malformations with the use of benzodiazepines during the first trimester of pregnancy. Pooled data from the case-controlled studies revealed a marginally significant two-fold increase in the risk of major malformations and oral cleft specifically. However, the case-controlled studies were heterogeneous, which decreases the results' reliability. Pooled data from the cohort studies, on the other hand, revealed no association between fetal exposure to benzodiazepines and the risk of oral clefts or any other major malformations.

The absolute risk for clefts, if present, remains small (i.e., the incidence of oral clefts in the general population is about one per thousand; the two-fold increase is therefore two per thousand).

Spontaneous abortion

No data are available on benzodiazepines and spontaneous abortion.

Neonatal effects

Babies exposed in utero to benzodiazepines should be watched carefully after birth for signs of abrupt discontinuation syndrome. This syndrome may include sedation, hypotonia, reluctance to suck, apnea, cyanosis and impaired metabolic responses to cold stress. The effects are self-limiting.

Long-term effects on the child

There have been no reports of long-term adverse effects on the intelligence quotient or neurodevelopment of children born to mothers who took benzodiazepines during pregnancy.

Breastfeeding

Most benzodiazepines are excreted into breast milk at low concentrations (less than five per cent of the maternal dose).[4] It is preferable to use the newer short-acting preparations (e.g., lorazepam) and avoid agents with a long half-life (e.g., diazepam); however, the short-acting benzodiazepines are more addictive.

Withdrawal effects on the mother

Women who suddenly stop taking a benzodiazepine may experience symptoms of abrupt discontinuation, including withdrawal symptoms or a re-emergence of the underlying illness. Symptoms may last for weeks or months and can occur when therapeutic doses are suddenly stopped. People who take benzodiazepines daily are at risk for withdrawal if they have been taking therapeutic doses for at least two months,[7] or excessive doses for at least two weeks.

Withdrawal symptoms start one to two days after short-acting benzodiazepines have been stopped and two to four days after long-acting benzodiazepines are discontinued. Symptoms commonly fall into two groups:

- anxiety-related symptoms—such as irritability, palpitations, panic attacks, labile mood, restlessness and insomnia
- neurological symptoms—including perceptual disturbances, primarily visual and auditory (e.g., sounds are unpleasantly loud, colours are harsh, staircases look longer than they actually are); odd sensations

such as depersonalization, derealization, déjà vu and dysperceptions; and seizures, psychosis and delirium.

These symptoms can last for many weeks. In addition, patients often report feeling fragile, with rapid shifts in emotions.

Effects of untreated illness

There are no definitive studies on the effect of untreated anxiety or insomnia in pregnancy or postpartum.

During all three trimesters of pregnancy it is normal for women to experience changes in sleep for a variety of reasons, including high hormone levels and physical changes. The greatest sleep disturbance is typically in the first month postpartum. This may increase the risk of postpartum depression and psychosis, though this hypothesis has not been studied extensively.[8]

One study compared the rates of major malformations between treated and untreated women with panic disorder. This study found a higher rate of isolated oral cleft and multiple congenital abnormalities in the children of mothers with the untreated panic disorder.[6] The authors concluded that anti-panic drug treatment appears to have a protective effect.

References

1. Health Canada. (2002). Anxiety disorders. In *A Report on Mental Illnesses in Canada*. Ottawa: Author. Available: www.mooddisorderscanada.ca/report/english/chapter4/index.htm. Accessed June 29, 2007.

2. Czeizel, A. (1987). Lack of evidence of teratogenicity of benzodiazepine drugs in Hungary. *Reproductive Toxicology, 1* (3), 183–188.

3. Bergman, U., Rosa, F.W., Baum, C., Wiholm, B.E. & Faich, G.A. (1992). Effects of exposure to benzodiazepine during fetal life. *Lancet, 340* (8821), 694–696.

4. McElhatton, P.R. (1994). The effects of benzodiazepine use during pregnancy and lactation. *Reproductive Toxicology, 8* (6), 461–475.

5. Dolovich, L.R., Addis, A., Vaillancourt, J.M., Power, J.D., Koren, G. & Einarson, T.R. (1998). Benzodiazepine use in pregnancy and major malformations or oral cleft: Meta-analysis of cohort and case-control studies. *British Medical Association Journal, 317* (7162), 839–843.

6. Acs, N., Banhidy, F., Horvath-Puho, E. & Czeizel, A.E. (2006). Maternal panic disorder and congenital abnormalities: A population-based case-control study. *Birth Defects Research. Part A, Clinical and Molecular Teratology, 76* (4), 253–261.

7. Kahan, M. & Wilson, L. (2002). *Managing Alcohol, Tobacco and Other Drug Problems: A Pocket Guide for Physicians and Nurses.* Toronto: Centre for Addiction and Mental Health.

8. Pien, G.W. & Schwab, R.J. (2004). Sleep disorders during pregnancy. *Sleep, 27* (7), 1405–1417.

Caffeine

Caffeine, the most commonly consumed stimulant in the world, is found in coffee, tea, chocolate, and some soft drinks, dietary aids, supplements and pain medications.

SUMMARY AND RECOMMENDATIONS

Women should be encouraged to monitor the amount of caffeine in food, drinks, supplements and pain medication throughout pregnancy, and to consume less than 150 milligrams of caffeine from all sources per day. Pregnant women consuming large amounts of caffeine should taper their use to this recommended level.

Caffeine content[1,2]

CAFFEINE SOURCE	AMOUNT
Coffee (8 oz / 227 mL) (many take-out coffee cup sizes are larger)	25–200 mg
Tea (8 oz / 227 mL)	40–120 mg
Cola and other soft drinks (12 oz / 341 mL)	25–75 mg
Energy drinks (17 oz / 483 mL)	100–600 mg
Chocolate (2 oz / 57 g)	10–35 mg

Fetal effects

During the first trimester, the half-life of caffeine remains at the normal rate of 2.5 to 4.5 hours. During the second and third trimesters, however, clearance is substantially delayed as the half-life extends to 10.5 hours.[3]

Caffeine is known to readily cross the placenta, and substantial quantities pass into the amniotic fluid and umbilical cord blood; it also appears in the urine and plasma of neonates. In addition, fetuses and neonates have low levels of the enzymes needed to metabolize caffeine, further increasing the half-life and, therefore, exposure to and possible accumulation of caffeine in their system.

Epidemiological studies[4] have produced incomplete or conflicting results about the effects of caffeine exposure in pregnancy.

Moderate caffeine consumption in pregnancy has not been associated with premature delivery or low birth weight.[5,6] A meta-analysis suggests a small but statistically significant increase in the risk of low-birth-weight babies in pregnant women who consume more than 150 milligrams of caffeine per day.[6]

Major malformations

Moderate caffeine consumption in pregnancy is not linked to any major malformations.

Spontaneous abortion

There are no known associations between moderate caffeine consumption in pregnancy and spontaneous abortion.

A small but statistically significant increase in the risk of spontaneous abortion has been found in pregnant women consuming a daily total of more than 150 milligrams of caffeine.[6] This conclusion is also supported by a study that found that extremely high levels of caffeine metabolite were associated with spontaneous abortion.[7]

Neonatal effects

In a small study, the newborns of women who consumed more than 500 milligrams of caffeine each day while pregnant showed cardiac arrhythmias, fine tremors and tachypnea.[8]

Long-term effects on the child

There are no reports of long-term effects on children due to in utero exposure to caffeine.

Breastfeeding

Caffeine is excreted into breast milk and reaches peak levels within one hour of maternal consumption; however, the amount of caffeine in breast milk is usually too low to show any significant effects. Nevertheless, large amounts of caffeine may accumulate and cause irritability and poor sleeping patterns in the baby.[9]

Withdrawal effects on the mother

Caffeine withdrawal symptoms can include headache, drowsiness, fatigue, decreased alertness, nausea and agitation.

Caffeine

References

1. Center for Science in the Public Interest. (n.d.). *Caffeine Content of Food and Drugs.* Washington, DC: Author. Available: www.cspinet.org/reports/caffeine.pdf. Accessed July 11, 2007.

2. Mayo Clinic. (2005). *Caffeine Content of Common Beverages.* Available: www.mayoclinic.com/health/caffeine/AN01211. Accessed July 11, 2007.

3. Knutti, R., Rothweiler, H. & Schlatter, C. (1982). The effect of pregnancy on the pharmacokinetics of caffeine. *Archives of Toxicology. Supplement, 5,* 187–192.

4. Koren, G. (2000). Caffeine during pregnancy? In moderation. *Canadian Family Physician, 46,* 801–803.

5. Linn, S., Schoenbaum, S.C., Monson, R.R., Rosner, B., Stubble-field, P.G. & Ryan, K.J. (1982). No association between coffee consumption and adverse outcomes of pregnancy. *New England Journal of Medicine, 306* (3), 141–145.

6. Fernandes, O., Shabarwal, M., Smiley, T., Pastuszak, A., Koren, G. & Einarson, T. (1998). Moderate to heavy caffeine consumption during pregnancy and relationship to spontaneous abortion and abnormal fetal growth: A meta-analysis. *Reproductive Toxicology, 12* (4), 435–444.

7. Klebanoff, M.A., Levine, R.J., Der Simonian, R., Clemens, J.D. & Wilkins, D.G. (1999). Maternal serum paraxanthine, a caffeine metabolite, and the risk of spontaneous abortion. *New England Journal of Medicine, 341* (22), 1639–1644.

8. Hadeed, A. & Siegel, S. (1993). Newborn cardiac arrhythmias associated with maternal caffeine use during pregnancy. *Clinical Pediatrics, 32* (1), 45–47.

9. Hill, R.M., Craig, J.P., Chaney, M.D., Tennyson, L.M. & McCulley, L.B. (1977). Utilization of over-the-counter drugs during pregnancy. *Clinical Obstetrics and Gynecology, 20* (2), 381–394.

Cannabis

Examples

Marijuana, hashish, hash oil, delta-9-tetrahydrocannabinol / cannabidiol (Sativex), delta-9-tetrahydrocannabinol (Marinol)

Street names

Marijuana: grass, weed, pot, dope (also used to refer to heroin), ganja, blunt, homegrown, reefer, bud, hydro, jay, spliff, Mary Jane (MJ), herb, doobie, simsemilla, chronic, bomb, joint

Hashish: hash

Hash oil: weed oil, honey oil

Cannabis is a drug prepared from the plant cannabis sativa, and can be smoked or ingested orally. It contains more than 400 chemicals, including delta-9-tetrahydrocannabinol (THC), the psychoactive component. When smoked, cannabis may pose some of the same risks associated with tobacco use.

Although cannabis is an illegal substance, in some circumstances a physician can prescribe its use through a Health Canada exemption. Clinical trials are done using government-grown cannabis, which is more standardized than cannabis sold on the street or grown in the home. Two legal pharmaceutical products containing THC are available in Canada.

SUMMARY AND RECOMMENDATIONS

- Cannabis use during pregnancy should be decreased or avoided altogether.
- Product monograms for Sativex and Marinol contraindicate the use of these products during pregnancy and breastfeeding.
- Cannabis appears to be excreted into breast milk in moderate amounts. Cannabis exposure through breast milk has not been shown to increase risk to the baby, but no appropriate confirming studies are available. Women who cannot stop using cannabinoids should discuss the risks of breastfeeding while using cannabis against the overall benefits of breastfeeding. Breast-feeding babies should be closely monitored.
- The effects of exposure to second-hand cannabis smoke in the baby's environment should also be considered.

Fetal effects

Studies have demonstrated a small reduction in birth weight associated with cannabis use during pregnancy. A meta-analysis of 10 studies on maternal cannabis use and birth weight shows only a weak association. For babies born to women who used any cannabis at all, the mean birth weight was 48 grams less than the mean birth weight of the babies in the control groups. For babies born to women who used cannabis at least four times a day, the mean birth weight was 131 grams less than the mean birth weight of babies in the control groups.[2]

Major malformations

Chemicals in cannabis, including THC, cross the placenta but cannabis has not been implicated as a human teratogen.[1]

Spontaneous abortion

Maternal cannabis use has not been associated with spontaneous abortion.

Neonatal effects

There are no reports of adverse neonatal effects resulting from a woman using cannabis during pregnancy.

Long-term effects on the child

Some studies have shown certain neurodevelopmental effects of prenatal exposure to cannabis; however, broader long-term developmental effects are unclear. In many studies, isolating the effect of cannabis from confounders (e.g., poverty, poor nutrition, unsafe housing, violence, the use of other drugs) is difficult.

Studies report that:

- at age three, sleep disturbances occurred in children of women who smoked cannabis during pregnancy.[3]

- at age 10, increased hyperactivity, impassivity, inattention and delinquency occurred in children from families with low-incomes exposed prenatally to cannabis.[4]

- from age nine to 12, no deficits in intelligence, memory or attention were reported, but poorer visual problem-solving skills were indicated in children exposed prenatally to cannabis (i.e., the hypothesis is that executive function is negatively affected).[5]

Breastfeeding

While the passage of cannabis into breast milk has not been studied extensively, cannabis appears to be excreted in moderate amounts. A 1982 study[6] found that 0.8 per cent of the maternal intake of one joint was ingested by an infant in one feeding. In women who used cannabis heavily, the milk-to-plasma ratio (i.e., levels in milk versus levels in maternal blood) was as high as 8:1.

THC is lipophilic and can accumulate in breast milk, theoretically affecting brain development. Possible effects on the baby include lethargy, less frequent and shorter feeding times, and decreased motor development at one year of age, particularly if exposure to cannabis was early in the post-partum period.[7] The long-term effects of using cannabis while breastfeeding are unclear.

Withdrawal effects on the mother

Symptoms of withdrawal from cannabis use, if they occur, are usually mild and may include sleep disturbance, irritability and loss of appetite. Symptomatic and supportive care for the mother is suggested.

Effects of untreated illness

In specific cases, cannabis and pharmaceutical products containing THC may be prescribed with a Health Canada exemption for symptomatic treatment of certain conditions (e.g., multiple sclerosis, AIDS, cancer). No studies have been completed of the continued use of cannabis during pregnancy under these conditions. The official product monographs for Marinol[8] and Sativex[9] contraindicate the use of these products during pregnancy and while breastfeeding. These products are used as symptomatic treatment, not to treat the underlying illness, and other standard treatments are available.

Also, cannabis has been suggested as a treatment for hyperemesis gravidarum, a serious and potentially fatal condition. In one study, women using cannabis during pregnancy reported a significant decrease in nausea, but not in vomiting.[10] In another study, 37 out of 40 women who used cannabis to treat "morning sickness" rated it either effective or extremely effective.[11]

References

1. Zuckerman, B., Frank, D.A., Hingson, R., Amaro, H., Levenson, S.M., Kayne, H. et al. (1989). Effects of maternal marijuana and cocaine use on fetal growth. *New England Journal of Medicine, 320* (12), 762–768.

2. English, D.R., Hulse, G.K., Milne, E., Holman, C.D. & Bower, C.I. (1997). Maternal cannabis use and birth weight: A meta-analysis. *Addiction, 92* (11), 1553–1560.

3. Dahl, R.E., Scher, M.S., Williamson, D.E., Robles, N. & Day, N. (1995). A longitudinal study of prenatal marijuana use: Effects on sleep and arousal at age three years. *Archives of Pediatrics and Adolescent Medicine, 149* (2), 145–150.

4. Goldschmidt, L., Day, N.L. & Richardson, G.A. (2000). Effects of prenatal marijuana exposure on child behavior problems at age 10. *Neurotoxicology and Teratology, 22* (3), 325–336.

5. Fried, P.A. & Watkinson, B. (2000). Visuoperceptual functioning differs in 9- to 12-year-olds prenatally exposed to cigarettes and marijuana. *Neurotoxicology and Teratology, 22* (1), 11–20.

6. Perez-Reyes, M. & Wall, M.E. (1982). Presence of delta9-tetrahydrocannabinol in human milk. *New England Journal of Medicine, 307* (13), 819–820.

7. Astley, S. & Little, R.E. (1990). Maternal marijuana use during lactation and infant development at one year. *Neurotoxicology and Teratology, 12* (2), 161–168.

8. Solvay Pharma. (2006). Marinol (delta-9-tetrahydrocannabinol): Product monograph. Markham, ON: Author.

9. Bayer Healthcare Pharmaceuticals. (2006). Sativex (delta-9-tetrahydrocannabinol / cannabidiol): Product monograph. Toronto: Author.

10. Chandra, K., Ho, E. Sarkar, M., Wolpin, J. & Koren, G. (2003). Characteristics of women using marijuana in pregnancy and their reported effects on symptoms of nausea and vomiting of pregnancy: A prospective controlled cohort study. *Journal of FAS International, 1*, e13

11. Westfall, R.E., Janssen, P.A., Lucas, P. & Capier, R. (2006). Survey of medicinal cannabis use among childbearing women: Patterns of its use in pregnancy and retroactive self-assessment of its efficacy against "morning sickness." *Complementary Therapies in Clinical Practice, 12*, 27–33.

Club drugs

Examples

3,4 methylenedioxymethamphetamine (ecstasy/MDMA); flunitrazepam (Rohypnol); gamma-hydroxybutyrate (GHB); ketamine

Street names

Ecstasy/MDMA: E, XTC, Adam, the love drug

Flunitrazepam (Rohypnol): roofies, roachies, La Roche, rope, ophies, ruffies

GHB: G, liquid ecstasy, liquid X, grievous bodily harm

Ketamine: special K, K, ket, vitamin K, cat tranquilizers

In recent years, certain drugs have emerged and become popular among young adults at dance clubs and raves— large all-night dance parties attended mainly by youth. Of what have come to be collectively termed "club drugs," MDMA is the most popular, and is often used concurrently with alcohol.

The only province-wide study that reports on ecstasy use in Canada is a 2005 Ontario student survey[1] in which 4.4 per cent of all students (ranging from 0.6 per cent of Grade 7 to 9.8 per cent of Grade 11 students) reported ecstasy use, a significant increase from 1993, when 0.6 per cent of students surveyed reported use.

There are no Canadian reports or studies on the prevalence of other club drug use.

SUMMARY AND RECOMMENDATIONS

- Since there is little information on the safety of club drugs, they should be avoided altogether during pregnancy and breastfeeding.

Fetal effects

Major malformations and spontaneous abortion

Of the few studies on the effects of club drugs, one prospective follow-up study of 136 babies exposed to MDMA in utero indicates that the drug may be associated with a significantly increased risk of congenital defects.[2] Twelve (8.8 per cent) of the 136 babies in the study had congenital malformations; however, there was no pattern of defects. The study did not include a comparison group, nor did it control for other possible contributing factors.

Another study reported data on 42 women who took club drugs in early pregnancy. There were three elective pregnancy terminations and two spontaneous abortions in this group. Of the 39 live-born babies, including one set of triplets, one baby had a congenital cardiac malformation. However, some of the mothers had used other substances while pregnant that could have harmed the fetus.[3]

Another study found no increased risk for major malformations or spontaneous abortions.[4]

Finally, another study of 54 women who had used MDMA during pregnancy compared birth outcomes with 54 unexposed women. No differences were reported in major malformations or spontaneous abortions.[5]

While there are no reports of fetal effects specific to flunitrazepam, it is a benzodiazepine and so there may be an increased risk of malformations, including oral cleft (see Benzodiazepines section, p. 65).

Neonatal effects

There are no reports of adverse neonatal effects in infants of mothers exposed to these drugs close to delivery.

The only published study on ketamine, when used as the sole anaesthetic during the induction-to-delivery period (i.e., in women at full term who are undergoing an elective caesarean section), reports that no adverse effects occurred in any of the exposed infants.[6]

Long-term effects on the child

There are no published studies of the long-term effects of club drug use during pregnancy.

Breastfeeding

There is no information on the effects of using any of these drugs while breastfeeding.

Withdrawal effects on the mother

Patterns of use of club drugs are generally different from those of other substances of abuse (i.e., use is not always daily or regular), and so physical dependence, tolerance and withdrawal are less likely.

Ecstacy: Physical withdrawal symptoms are not usually reported; however, after the drug's effects wear off there have been reports of symptoms similar to a depressive episode.[7]

Flunitrazepam: See Benzodiazepines section, p. 65.

GHB: Stopping regular use abruptly can result in anxiety, tremors, insomnia and other unpleasant, potentially dangerous side-effects, including paranoia with hallucinations and high blood pressure.[8]

Ketamine: Withdrawal effects have not been reported.

References

1. Adlaf, E. & Paglia-Boak, A. (2005). *Drug Use among Ontario Students, 1997–2005: 2005 Ontario Student Drug Use Survey (OSDUS)*—Highlights (CAMH Research Document Series No. 17). Available: www.camh.net/News_events/News_releases_and_media_advisories_and_backgrounders/osdus2005_highlights.html. Accessed June 29, 2007.

2. McElhatton, P.R., Bateman, D.N., Evans, C., Pughe, K.R. & Thomas, S.H. (1999). Congenital anomalies after prenatal ecstasy exposure. *Lancet, 354* (9188), 1441–1442.

3. van Tonningen-van Driel, M.M., Garbis-Berkvens, J.M. & Reuvers-Lodewijks, W.E. (1999). Pregnancy outcome after ecstasy use: 43 cases followed by the Teratology Information Service of the National Institute for Public Health and Environment (RIVM). *Nederlands Tijdschrift Voor Geneeskunde, 143* (1), 27–31.

4. Smith, L.M., LaGasse, L.L., Derauf, C., Grant, P., Shah, R., Arria, A. et al. (2006). The infant development, environment, and lifestyle study: Effects of prenatal methamphetamine exposure, polydrug exposure, and poverty on intrauterine growth. *Pediatrics, 118* (3), 1149–1156.

5. Sarkar, M. (2006, June). *Pregnancy Outcome of Women Exposed to MDMA.* Abstract presented at the meeting of the Organization of Teratology Information Services, Tucson, AZ.

6. Baraka, A., Louis, F. & Dalleh, R. (1990). Maternal awareness and neonatal outcome after ketamine induction of anaesthesia for caesarean section. *Canadian Journal of Anaesthesia, 37* (6), 641–644.

7. Huxster, J.K., Pirona, A. & Morgan, M.J. (2006). The sub-acute effects of recreational ecstasy (MDMA) use: A controlled study in humans. *Journal of Psychopharmacology. 20* (2), 281–290.

8. Gonzalez, A. & Nutt, D.J. (2005). Gamma hydroxy butyrate abuse and dependency. *Journal of Psychopharmacology 9* (2), 195–204.

Cocaine

Street names

Blow, C, coke, dust, flake, powder lines, snow

Crack cocaine: freebase, rock

Cocaine is a stimulant that readily crosses the placenta.[1] Cocaine hydrochloride, a white crystalline powder, can be snorted or injected. Powder cocaine can also be chemically changed to create crystals or "rocks"—known as "freebase" or "crack"—that can be smoked.

Most women who use cocaine use at least one other drug (e.g., alcohol, tobacco, cannabis)[2] and have other risk factors related to poor pregnancy outcome, including poor nutrition, high gravidity and lack of prenatal care.[3]

SUMMARY AND RECOMMENDATIONS

- Abstinence from cocaine use throughout pregnancy is recommended. However, discontinuing cocaine at any time during pregnancy can improve the fetal outcome.

- Careful monitoring of neonates is recommended; comfort measures, especially touch, reduced stimulation (e.g., a quiet room with dim lighting, no excessive testing, keeping interventions to a minimum) and breastfeeding, are generally sufficient.

- Breastfeeding while using cocaine is not recommended. If a woman uses cocaine, she should not breastfeed within three days of using the drug (i.e., she should pump and discard the milk). The risks of breastfeeding while using cocaine must be weighed against the overall benefits of breastfeeding.

Fetal effects

Women who use cocaine during pregnancy are more likely than those who do not use the drug to have placental abruption (which may cause fetal hypoxia and ischemia) and preterm premature rupture of membranes.[3] When cocaine crosses the placenta into the fetus's circulation, fetal hypertension and increased cardiac output could also increase the risk of intracranial lesions and hemorrhage.[1]

An infant prenatally exposed to cocaine is more likely than non-exposed infants to be born prematurely and to have intrauterine growth retardation (IUGR), lower birth weight and a smaller head circumference.[4-6]

In addition, the combination of cocaine with other fetotoxins (e.g., cigarette smoke and/or alcohol) may result in a negative synergistic effect. For example, one study found that the percentage of babies weighing less than 2,500 grams at birth (i.e., low birth weight) was significantly higher among mothers who combined cocaine and cigarettes (50 per cent) than among those who used cocaine alone (eight per cent). Also, the infants exposed n utero to cocaine and tobacco were, on average, 500 grams smaller than those exposed to cocaine alone.[7]

Another study[8] compared three groups of women: one group used cocaine throughout pregnancy, a second group used cocaine during the first trimester only and a third group did not use cocaine at all. Women who used cocaine in only the first trimester experienced placental abruption more frequently than women who did not use cocaine at all, but had similar rates of preterm delivery and low-birth-weight and IUGR infants to those of women who did not use cocaine. The effects of use were more significant in the women who used cocaine throughout their pregnancies—they were significantly more likely (25 per cent) than the drug-free controls (five per cent) to deliver low-birth-weight infants.[8]

Major malformations

While there is no established cause-and-effect relationship between prenatal cocaine exposure and increased major malformations, there is enough evidence to suggest that cocaine use during pregnancy is a significant concern for maternal and fetal effects.[9] A meta-analysis[10] of 20 papers compared (i) women who used only cocaine versus a control group of women who did not use substances, (ii) women with polysubstance use involving cocaine versus a control group of women who did not use substances and (iii) women with polysubstance use that included cocaine versus women with polysubstance use that did not include cocaine. The meta-analysis found a significantly greater likelihood of neonatal genitourinary malformations in cocaine-exposed infants,[10] which appears to be dose related.[11] Other studies[9,12] did not observe any other congenital abnormalities in cocaine-exposed infants.

Spontaneous abortion

A meta-analysis reported an increase in spontaneous abortions in women who used cocaine, even when there was control for polysubstance use.[10]

Neonatal effects

Infants exposed in utero to cocaine may have significant neurobehavioural impairments during the neonatal period; they usually occur on days two and three.[13] An increased degree of irritability, tremulousness and muscular rigidity have been observed; gastrointestinal symptoms (e.g., vomiting, diarrhea) and seizures have also been reported.[12] All of these effects seem to be more consistent with cocaine exposure rather than with cocaine withdrawal.[13,14]

Long-term effects on the child

Long-term effects of maternal cocaine use on children are not known. Language delays (i.e., delays in expressive and verbal comprehension) and behavioural problems may be encountered at school.[15,16] Two primary risk factors that are also associated with cocaine use are poor maternal functioning and an inadequate caring environment.[17]

One study[18] followed children of 28 women who reported light to moderate cocaine use (i.e., an average of 3.3 grams per month [approximately 3.7 lines per day]) during their first trimester. The children were examined at delivery and at eight months, 18 months, three years and six years of age. The comparison group consisted of 523 women who used no cocaine for the entire duration of the study as well as the year before pregnancy. The study only reported on the status of the children at the six-year mark, at which time no significant effects of prenatal cocaine exposure on growth, intellectual ability, academic achievement or teacher-rated classroom behaviour were reported. (Note: More of the women in this study who used cocaine were working or attending school; their monthly income was also higher than the income of those in the comparison group.)

A more recent study showed that potential long-term risks for the child are more closely related to low birth weight and the environmental risks associated with cocaine exposure in the caregiving environment, than to cocaine exposure itself.[9]

Breastfeeding

Cocaine passes into breast milk, and both powder cocaine and crack have been known to cause the baby to experience irritability, trembling, vomiting, diarrhea and seizures.[12] However, there are no known data to confirm this and the percentage dose in breast milk is unknown.

Withdrawal effects on the mother

About 10 per cent of people who use cocaine meet the diagnostic criteria for cocaine dependence.[19] Symptoms of withdrawal may include fatigue, nightmares, insomnia, increased appetite, anxiety, psychomotor agitation or retardation, and dysphoric mood. Withdrawal from cocaine is primarily a psychological process, and can be safely undertaken. Women should be provided supportive care and monitored for suicidal ideation.

People who have been bingeing on cocaine will sometimes sleep heavily for one or two days after the binge. They may then experience several weeks or months of depression and insomnia, with vivid dreams and strong cravings for cocaine. Medical treatments have not yet been shown to be effective for cocaine withdrawal or cravings.

References

1. Plessinger, M.A. & Woods, J.R. (1998). Cocaine in pregnancy: Recent data on maternal and fetal risks. *Obstetrics and Gynecology Clinics of North America, 25* (1), 99–118.

2. Gingras, J.L. & O'Donnell, K. (1998). State control in the substance-exposed fetus. I. The fetal neurobehavioral profile: An assessment of fetal state, arousal, and regulation competency. *Annals of the New York Academy of Sciences, 846,* 262–276.

3. Sprauve, M.E., Lindsay, M.K., Herbert, S. & Graves, W. (1997). Adverse perinatal outcome in parturients who use crack cocaine. *Obstetrics & Gynecology, 89* (5 Pt. 1), 674–678.

4. Kliegman, R.M., Madura, D. & Kiwi, R. (1994). Relation of maternal cocaine use to the risks of prematurity and low birth weight. *Journal of Pediatrics, 124* (5 Pt. 1), 751–756.

5. Bateman, D.A., Ng, S.K., Hansen, C.A. & Heagarty, M.C. (1993). The effects of intrauterine cocaine exposure in newborns. *American Journal of Public Health, 83* (2), 190–193.

6. Eyler, F.D., Behnke, M., Conlon, M., Woods, N.S. & Frentzen, B. (1994). Prenatal cocaine use: A comparison of neonates matched on maternal risk factors. *Neurotoxicology and Teratology, 16* (1), 81–87.

7. Forman, R., Klein, J., Meta, D., Barks, J., Greenwald, M. & Koren, G. (1993). Maternal and neonatal characteristics following exposure to cocaine in Toronto. *Reproductive Toxicology, 7* (6), 619–622.

8. Chasnoff, I.J., Griffith, D.R., MacGregor, S., Dirkes, K. & Burns, K.A. (1989). Temporal patterns of cocaine use in pregnancy: Perinatal outcome. *Journal of the American Medical Association, 261* (12), 1741–1744.

9. Messinger, D.S., Bauer, C.R., Das, A., Seifer, R., Lester, B.M., Lagasse, L.L. et al. (2004). The maternal lifestyle study: Cognitive motor and behavioral outcomes of cocaine-exposed and opiate-exposed infants through three years of age. *Pediatrics, 113* (6) 1677–1685.

10. Lutiger, B., Graham, K., Einarson, T.R. & Koren, G. (1991). Relationship between gestational cocaine use and pregnancy outcome: A meta-analysis. *Teratology, 44* (4), 405–414.

11. Chiriboga, C.A., Brust, J.C., Bateman, D. & Hauser, W.A. (1999). Dose-response effect of fetal cocaine exposure on newborn neurologic function. *Pediatrics, 103* (1), 79–85.

12. Briggs, G.G., Freeman, R.K. & Yaffe, S.J. (2002). *Drugs in Pregnancy and Lactation: A Reference Guide to Fetal and Neonatal Risk* (6th ed.). Philadelphia, PA: Lippincott Williams & Wilkins.

13. American Academy of Pediatrics Committee on Drugs. (1998). Neonatal drug withdrawal. *Pediatrics, 101* (6), 1079–1088.

14. Bauer, C.R., Langer, J.L., Shankaran, S., Bada, H.S., Lester, B., Wright, L. et al. (2005). Acute neonatal effects of cocaine exposure during pregnancy. *Archives of Pediatrics and Adolescent Medicine, 159* (9), 824–834.

15. Delaney-Black, V., Covington, C., Templin, T., Kershaw, T., Nordstrom-Klee, B., Ager, J. et al. (2000). Expressive language development of children exposed to cocaine prenatally: Literature review and report of a prospective cohort study. *Journal of Communication Disorders, 33* (6), 463–480; Quiz 480–481.

16. Nulman, I., Rovet, J., Greenbaum, R., Loebstein, M., Wolpin, J., Pace-Asciak, P. et al. (2001). Neurodevelopment of adopted children exposed in utero to cocaine: The Toronto Adoption Study. *Clinical and Investigative Medicine, 24* (3), 129–137.

17. Lester, B.M. (2000). Prenatal cocaine exposure and child outcome: A model for the study of the infant at risk. *The Israel Journal of Psychiatry and Related Sciences, 37* (3), 223–235.

18. Richardson, G.A., Conroy, M.L. & Day, N.L. (1996). Prenatal cocaine exposure: Effects on the development of school-age children. *Neurotoxicology and Teratology, 18* (6), 627–634.

19. O'Grady, C.P. & Skinner, W.J.W. (2007). *A Family Guide to Concurrent Disorders.* Toronto: Centre for Addiction and Mental Health.

Inhalants

Examples

Solvents (e.g., cleaning fluids, felt tip markers, gasoline, glue, paint thinners, room odourizers, VCR head cleaner), nitrites (e.g., room odourizers, VCR head cleaner), nitrous oxide

Street names

Solvents: sniff

Nitrites: poppers, some sold under "brand" names such as Rush, Bolt, Kix

Nitrous oxide: whippets

Inhalants are chemical vapours or gases that can be sniffed (inhaled directly from the container), "bagged" (inhaled from a bag) or "huffed" (inhaled from a soaked rag held to the face). Inhalants (many of which are volatile solvents) usually take effect within minutes and produce an alcohol-like effect, but with more distortion of perception (i.e., of the shape, size and colour of objects, and of time and space).

SUMMARY AND RECOMMENDATIONS

- Women should avoid using inhalants during pregnancy.
- Women who use inhalants after childbirth risk these substances entering the breast milk and risk passive exposure of the baby to the substances. They should therefore refrain from breastfeeding while using inhalants.

Fetal effects

Several case reports and animal studies have demonstrated a reduction in birth weight associated with the use of inhalants in pregnancy.[1,2]

Major malformations

While teratogenicity due to occupational exposure to organic solvents (i.e., relatively long-term exposure to lower concentrations) has been studied, the teratogenic potential of organic solvent abuse has not been comprehensively examined. In a meta-analysis of 10 studies of maternal solvent exposure, five showed major malformations.[3] Several case reports and animal studies demonstrate that brief, repeated, prenatal exposure to high concentrations of organic solvents can cause neurodevelopmental delay and facial abnormalities similar to fetal alcohol syndrome.[1,2]

Spontaneous abortion

In a meta-analysis of 10 studies of maternal solvent exposure, five showed an increased risk for spontaneous abortion.[3]

Neonatal effects

In a study of 50 babies born to women abusing solvents, 24 babies showed neonatal abstinence syndrome.[2]

Long-term effects on the child

The long-term effects on the child are not clear; however, there is some evidence that prenatal exposure may cause long-term neurodevelopmental impairments, such as deficits in cognitive, speech and motor skills.[1]

Breastfeeding

The passage of inhalants into breast milk has not been extensively studied.

Withdrawal effects on the mother

Withdrawal symptoms for inhalants are similar to those for alcohol withdrawal, and may include insomnia, tremors, nausea, extreme confusion, anxiety and seizures.

References

1. Jones, H.E. & Balster, R.L. (1998). Inhalant abuse in pregnancy. *Obstetrics and Gynecology Clinics of North America, 25* (1), 153–167.

2. Scheeres, J.J. & Chudley, A.E. (2002). Solvent abuse in pregnancy: A perinatal perspective. *Journal of Obstetrics and Gynaecology Canada, 24* (1), 22–26.

3. McMartin, K.I., Chu, M., Kopecky, E., Einarson, T.R. & Koren, G. (1998). Pregnancy outcome following maternal organic solvent exposure: A meta-analysis of epidemiologic studies. *American Journal of Industrial Medicine, 34* (3), 288–292.

Lithium

Examples

Carbolith, Duralith, Lithane, Lithizine

Lithium is an anti-manic medication used to treat bipolar disorder,* which affects more than 444,000 (2.6%) Canadians between 25 and 64 years of age.[1]

Bipolar disorder usually begins in late adolescence and often first appears as depression during the teenage years, though it can also begin in early childhood or later in life. An equal number of men and women develop the illness, which is found among all ages, races, ethnic groups and social classes. A significant number of women of childbearing age suffer from bipolar disorder and may therefore require treatment with lithium.

Early information about the teratogenic risk associated with lithium exposure during pregnancy came from biased retrospective reports.[2] More recent epidemiological data indicates that the risk is much lower than previously suggested.[3]

SUMMARY AND RECOMMENDATIONS

- A level II ultrasound and fetal echocardiogram can be performed at 16 to 18 weeks gestation to rule out cardiac anomalies.

*Lithium can also be used as adjunct therapy for several other treatment-refractory disorders.

- Toxic effects can be minimized by monitoring serum lithium levels and keeping minimally effective plasma levels throughout gestation, particularly during the last month of pregnancy. In addition, briefly suspending lithium therapy prior to delivery can reduce perinatal complications. Specialized pediatric personnel should be available at the time of delivery, especially for women on high doses.

- Suspending therapy in the first trimester of pregnancy may be an option for some women with mild to moderate illness, or for women with a long history of euthymia during pre-pregnancy treatment. However, treatment should be reintroduced either in later pregnancy or immediately postpartum.

- The newborn should be monitored carefully for possible lithium toxicity, which can include cyanosis, hypotonia, bradycardia, thyroid depression with goitre, atrial flutter, cardiomegaly, hepatomegaly and diabetes insipidus. These toxic effects are usually self-limiting and resolve upon renal excretion of the drug within one to two weeks.

- Women who are committed to breastfeeding need to be informed that therapeutic drug monitoring of lithium in their breast milk and/or in their infant's blood (e.g., regular blood tests), coupled with close monitoring of adverse effects, will be necessary as long as they continue to breastfeed.

Fetal effects

Lithium has been associated with an increase in birth weight.[4]

Major malformations

By 1983, the International Registry of Lithium-Exposed Babies reported a total of 225 cases of children whose mothers who took lithium while pregnant.[2] Evaluation of the registry at that time revealed that the number of cases of Ebstein's anomaly far exceeded the spontaneous occurrence in the general population. However, there were no population-based, prospective, controlled studies to compare the occurrence rate of Ebstein's or to ascertain the actual incidence.

In 1992, one study recruited and followed 148 women who took lithium during their first trimester. Pregnancy outcome was compared with that of controls, who were matched for maternal age. Rates of major congenital malformations did not differ between the lithium (2.8 per cent) and control (2.4 per cent) groups. One woman in the lithium group chose to terminate her pregnancy after a prenatal echocardiogram detected Ebstein's anomaly.[3]

In another cohort of 59 children who had been exposed to lithium in utero, four (i.e., 6.8 per cent) had congenital heart disease but none had Ebstein's anomaly.[5] In a case-control study of children with cardiac defects, including 25 cases of Ebstein's anomaly, none of the mothers had been exposed to lithium.[6]

These results appear to indicate that lithium is not a major human teratogen, and that the risk for Ebstein's anomaly is 0.05 per cent (i.e., one in 2,000) for babies whose mothers take lithium during pregnancy. A further review—upon analysis of the results of various cohort, prospective and retrospective studies and a small number of case reports—indicates that lithium is a "weak" human teratogen. The malformations mainly attributable to lithium are cardiac defects. There is a possibility that lithium may be associated with Ebstein's anomaly, but present evidence cannot definitely confirm or rule out this connection.[4,7]

Spontaneous abortion

No studies have examined whether lithium use results in an increased risk for spontaneous abortion.

Neonatal effects

Lithium completely equilibrates across the placenta. Higher lithium levels at the time of delivery are associated with increased perinatal complications.[8] Specifically, a review of the literature published from 1978 to 2004 identifies 30 babies (with adequate clinical description) who were exposed to lithium during gestation. A substantial number of these babies presented with neurodevelopmental deficits and depressed neurological status during the neonatal period, including hypotonia, respiratory distress syndrome, cyanosis, lethargy, and weak suck and Moro reflexes. The majority of these adverse effects resolved and most babies made a full recovery.[4]

Long-term effects on the child

There are no reports of long-term effects on children whose mothers took lithium during pregnancy.

Breastfeeding

In the past, lithium has typically been contraindicated for use in lactating women because of early reports suggesting high excretion into breast milk. A relatively recent study conducted to ascertain the excretion of lithium into human milk and to assess infant safety after breastfeeding found that lithium excretion in breast milk varies widely (from zero to 30 per cent of the maternal dose) from woman to woman.[9]

Withdrawal effects on the mother

Several reports have documented symptoms of abrupt discontinuation of lithium (e.g., rapid reoccurrence of mania). One review described 14 people who discontinued lithium abruptly, seven of whom subsequently became manic within 13 to 19 days. This review also identified

depression and suicidal behaviour in the participants.[10] Another study stated that three of 18 participants studied relapsed within four days of lithium being abruptly discontinued; several others exhibited hand tremors, polyuria, general muscular weakness, polydipsia and dry mouth.[11]

Effects of untreated illness

Pregnancy does not protect against mood fluctuations in untreated women. Maintenance of euthymia during pregnancy is critical because relapse during this period strongly predicts a difficult postpartum course.

One study comparing pregnant and non-pregnant women with bipolar disorder found similar rates of recurrence after discontinuation of lithium in the first 40 weeks, but the pregnant women had a high risk of recurrence during the postpartum period.[12]

References

1. Wilkins, K. (2004). Bipolar I disorder, social support and work. *Supplement to Health Reports, 15,* 23–41. Ottawa: Statistics Canada. (Catalogue No. 82-003)

2. Linden, S. & Rich, C.L. (1983). The use of lithium during pregnancy and lactation. *Journal of Clinical Psychiatry, 44* (10), 358–361.

3. Jacobson, S.J., Jones, K., Johnson, K., Ceolin, L., Kaur, P., Sahn, D. et al. (1992). Prospective multicentre study of pregnancy outcome after lithium exposure during first trimester. *Lancet, 339* (8792), 530–533.

4. Giles, J.J. & Bannigan, J.G. (2006). Teratogenic and developmental effects of lithium [Review]. *Current Pharmaceutical Design, 12* (12), 1531–1541.

5. Warkany, J. (1988). Teratogen update: Lithium. *Teratology, 38* (6), 593–597.

6. Källén, B. & Tandberg, A., (1983). Lithium and pregnancy. A cohort study on manic-depressive women. *Acta Psychiatrica Scandinavica, 68* (2), 134–139.

7. Cohen, L.S., Friedman, J.M., Jefferson, J.W., Johnson, E.M. & Weiner, M.L. (1994). A re-evaluation of risk of in utero exposure to lithium. *Journal of the American Medical Association, 271* (123), 1828–1829.

8. Newport, D.J., Viguera, A.C., Beach, A.J., Ritchie, J.C., Cohen, L.S. & Stowe, Z.N. (2005). Lithium placental passage and obstetrical outcome: Implications for clinical management during late pregnancy. *American Journal of Psychiatry, 162* (11), 2162–2170.

9. Moretti, M.E., Koren, G., Verjee, Z. & Ito, S. (2003). Monitoring lithium in breast milk: An individualized approach for breast-feeding mothers. *Therapeutic Drug Monitoring, 25* (3), 364–366.

10. Mander, A.J. & Loudon, J.B. (1988). Rapid recurrence of mania following abrupt discontinuation of lithium. *Lancet, 2* (8601), 15–17.

11. Baldessarini, R.J., Suppes, T. & Tondo, L. (1996). Lithium withdrawal in bipolar disorder: Implications for clinical practice and experimental therapeutics research. *American Journal of Therapeutics, 3* (7), 492–496.

12. Viguera, A.C., Nonacs, R., Cohen, L.S., Tondo, L., Murray, A. & Baldessarini, R.J. (2000). Risk of recurrence of bipolar disorder in pregnant and nonpregnant women after discontinuing lithium maintenance. *American Journal of Psychiatry, 157* (2), 179–184.

Opioids

Examples

Codeine (in Tylenol 3), heroin, hydrocodone (Tussionex), hydromorphone (Dilaudid), meperidine (Demerol), methadone, morphine (MS Contin, Statex), oxycodone (Percodan, Percocet, OxyContin)

Street names

Heroin: junk, H, smack, horse, skag, dope (also used to refer to cannabis), shit

Morphine: M, morph, Miss Emma

Methadone: juice, meth (also used to refer to methamphetamine)

Hydromorphone (Dilaudid): juice

Oxycodone: oxy, OC, percs

Opioids are used therapeutically for the treatment of pain and recreationally for their psychogenic qualities. Opioids can also be used to control coughs and diarrhea, or for treating addiction (i.e., to other opioids). While these drugs occur naturally (e.g., morphine), some are produced semi-synthetically (e.g., heroin) or synthetically (e.g., methadone).

All opioids produce morphine-like effects; however, since they also produce feelings of euphoria, they can be prone to abuse. Opioids are taken orally, injected or smoked. Their use can range from occasional (e.g., over-the-counter codeine) to daily, prescribed use to various forms of abuse. Injection opioid use with unsterile needles increases the risk of serious infection (e.g., hepatitis, HIV) in both the mother and the fetus or baby.

SUMMARY AND RECOMMENDATIONS

- Women who take moderate doses of prescribed opioids (e.g., Tylenol 3, three to four tablets daily), who are not psychologically or physically dependent on the drug and who become pregnant may continue with the medication, but at the lowest effective dose possible.

- If tapering is considered, it should be the woman's choice and she should be under close supervision. Dose reductions should be limited to no more than 10 per cent of the total dose per week. Tapering should start in the second trimester (i.e., 14 to 28 weeks) to reduce risk of spontaneous abortion or preterm labour. In addition, a pain expert and addiction medicine specialist may provide helpful support during pregnancy.

- Methadone is safer to use during pregnancy than are illegal opioids, and is the standard of care for opioid dependence. Methadone maintenance treatment reduces opioid withdrawal and thus improves maternal health and compliance with prenatal care, which in turn reduces fetal and neonatal complications. Only physicians experienced in methadone use should prescribe the drug, since dose requirements must be closely monitored and may change during the pregnancy.

- Neonates of mothers treated with methadone should be observed in hospital for symptoms of withdrawal for at least four to five days.
- Women who take methadone can safely breastfeed their babies; very small amounts of methadone are present in breast milk.[1]
- Suggestions for prescribing codeine to women who are breastfeeding include prescribing for two to three days only to prevent neonatal accumulation of morphine, counselling parents to watch for signs of overdose in their babies and following up closely with breastfed infants who have symptoms such as excessive drowsiness.[2]

Fetal effects

Opioid withdrawal in the third trimester can lead to premature labour.[3]

Major malformations

Opioids (including heroin) are not linked to any major malformations.[4,5]

In the late 1970s and early 1980s, a few studies suggested that opioid abuse in the first and second trimesters may slightly increase the risk of some malformations (e.g., inguinal hernias, and cleft lip and palate). However, study confounders—such as the mother's use of multiple drugs, maternal disease, lack of prenatal care, poverty and malnutrition—make it impossible to form definite conclusions about this increased risk from these early studies.[6–8] More recent studies that control for these confounders have not found an increased risk of major malformations.[9]

Spontaneous abortion

Occasional prescribed use of opioids is generally considered safe. However, when used regularly (e.g., on a daily basis), opioids can increase the risk of spontaneous abortion.[10] In addition, opioid withdrawal can trigger uterine contractions in the first trimester that can lead to spontaneous abortion.[3]

Neonatal effects

In general, a neonate experiences withdrawal only when the mother used opioids regularly during pregnancy. Forty to 60 per cent of infants born to women using heroin, and up to 85 per cent of those born to mothers taking methadone, experience withdrawal.[3]

In a newborn, withdrawal is difficult to diagnose if the mother does not disclose her opioid use because other newborn conditions (e.g., hypoglycemia) have similar symptoms. Withdrawal usually begins shortly after birth, typically within 24 hours but possibly up to two weeks ater, depending on the half-life of the opioid. Withdrawal can last for several weeks, and symptoms include difficulty breathing upon birth and extreme drowsiness. Poor feeding, irritability, sweating, tremors, vomiting and diarrhea may also occur, while seizures and death have been reported in severe, untreated withdrawal cases. Babies undergoing opioid withdrawal commonly experience a more severe withdrawal if the mother is also taking alcohol or benzodiazepines.

Treatment of the baby's withdrawal from opioids consists primarily of supportive care and may include the administration of small doses of morphine.

Neonatal withdrawal is not associated with any long-term complications.

Long-term effects on the child

Babies of mothers who use heroin present with some long-term effects. One study found that at three to six years of age, for example, children whose mothers were addicted to heroin were lower in weight and height compared to the control group, and impaired in behavioural, perceptual and organizational abilities compared to the controls.[11]

Breastfeeding

At therapeutic doses, most opioids (e.g., morphine, meperidine, methadone) are excreted into breast milk in minimal amounts and are, therefore, compatible with breastfeeding.[1,12,13] These levels are generally considered unlikely to prevent withdrawal in neonates, although one study found that there was less need for neonatal abstinence syndrome treatment in breastfed infants than in those fed with formula.[14] This may be due in part to factors related to the breastfeeding itself rather than the opioid in the breast milk.[15]

For mothers being treated with methadone, the amount that passes into the milk is small (two to four per cent).[16] In its 1994 guidelines,[17] the American Academy of Pediatrics (AAP) recommended breastfeeding only at maternal doses of 20 milligrams or less. Since then, there have been reports of maternal methadone doses of up to 180 milligrams during breastfeeding without adverse effects.[18–21] The 2001 AAP guidelines eliminated the dose restriction, and methadone is now considered compatible with breastfeeding.[22]

Codeine is considered compatible with breastfeeding by most standard references and the AAP,[22] but a recent case report has brought this recommendation into question. A baby who had been breastfed by a mother who was taking codeine for postlabour pain died from morphine overdose 13 days after birth.[23] It was later determined that the mother was an ultrarapid metabolizer with the enzyme cytochrome P450 2D6, and produced much more morphine than most mothers would. Thus far, no new recommendations have emerged. Though ultrarapid metabolizers are rare, the frequency of codeine prescriptions postpartum raises concern. Suggestions include prescribing for two to three days only to prevent neonatal accumulation of morphine, counselling parents to watch for signs of overdose in their babies and following up closely with breastfed infants who have symptoms such as excessive drowsiness.[2]

Withdrawal effects on the mother

Opioid withdrawal symptoms include nausea, vomiting, diarrhea, sweating, myalgias, chills, rhinorrhea, runny eyes and piloerection. Psychological symptoms can include insomnia, anxiety, strong drug cravings and dysphoria.[24]

Pregnancy-specific opioid withdrawal symptoms include abdominal cramping and uterine irritability, which may lead to an increased risk of spontaneous abortion, preterm labour, fetal hypoxia and fetal death.[24]

Withdrawal symptoms begin six to 24 hours after the last opioid dose, depending on the opioid's duration of action.

Patients in severe withdrawal may appear anxious and uncomfortable. They may be huddled over, with chills and vomiting. Physical symptoms peak at two to three days, and largely resolve in five to 10 days. Psychological symptoms (e.g., insomnia, anxiety, cravings) may persist for weeks or months.[24] Patients typically find the psychological symptoms of opioid withdrawal far more disturbing than the physical withdrawal symptoms.

For adults, the main complications of opioid withdrawal are suicidality and overdose.[24] Suicide attempts may occur in settings where a person is unable to obtain relief from the withdrawal experience (e.g., a prison). People who stop using opioids begin to lose their tolerance to the drug within days. As a result, if they relapse and begin taking their usual opioid dose again, they may be at risk for overdose.

References

1. Wojnar-Horton, R.E., Kristensen, J.H., Yapp, P., Ilett, K.F., Dusci, L.J. & Hackett, L.P. (1997). Methadone distribution and excretion into breast milk of clients in a methadone maintenance programme. *British Journal of Clinical Pharmacology, 44* (6), 543–547.

2. Madadi, P., Koren, G., Cairns, J., Chitayat, D., Gaedigk, A., Leeder, J.S. et al. (2007). Safety of codeine during breastfeeding. *Canadian Family Physician, 53,* 33–25.

3. Bell, G.L. & Lau, K. (1995). Perinatal and neonatal issues of substance abuse. *Pediatric Clinics of North America, 42* (2), 261–281.

4. Heinonen, O.P., Slone, D. & Shapiro, S. (1977). *Birth Defects and Drugs in Pregnancy.* Littleton, MA: Publishing Sciences Group.

5. Little, B.B., Snell, L.M., Klein, V.R., Gilstrap, L.C., Knoll, K.A. & Breckenridge, J.D. (1990). Maternal and fetal effects of heroin addiction during pregnancy. *Journal of Reproductive Medicine, 35* (2), 159–162.

6. Bracken, M.B. & Holford, T.R. (1981). Exposure to prescribed drugs in pregnancy and association with congenital malformations. *Obstetrics and Gynecology, 58* (3), 336–344.

7. Saxen, I. (1975). Associations between oral clefts and drugs taken during pregnancy. *International Journal of Epidemiology, 4* (1), 37–44.

8. Saxen, I. (1975). Epidemiology of cleft lip and palate: An attempt to rule out chance correlations. *British Journal of Preventative Social Medicine, 29* (2), 103–110.

9. Messinger, D.S., Bauer, C.R., Das, A., Seifer, R., Lester, B.M., Lagasse, L.L. et al. (2004). The maternal lifestyle study: Cognitive, motor, and behavioral outcomes of cocaine-exposed and opiate-exposed infants through three years of age. *Pediatrics 113* (6), 1677–1685.

10. Kaltenbach, K., Berghella, V. & Finnegan, L. (1998). Opioid dependence during pregnancy: Effects and management. *Obstetrics and Gynecology Clinics of North America, 25* (1), 139–151.

11. Wilson, G.S., McCreary, R., Kean, J. & Baxter, J.C. (1979). The development of preschool children of heroin-addicted mothers: A controlled study. *Pediatrics, 63* (1), 135–141.

12. Feiberg, V.L., Rosenborg, D., Broen, C.C. & Mogensen, J.V. (1989). Excretion of morphine in human breast milk. *Acta Anaesthesiologica Scandinavica, 33* (5), 426–428.

13. Robieux, I., Koren, G., Vandenbergh, H. & Schneiderman, J. (1990). Morphine excretion in breast milk and resultant exposure of a nursing infant. *Journal of Toxicology Clinical Toxicology, 28* (3), 365–370.

14. Abdel-Latif, M.E., Pinner, J., Clews, S., Cooke, F., Lui, K. & Oei, J. (2006). Effects of breast milk on the severity and outcome of neonatal abstinence syndrome among infants of drug-dependent mothers. *Pediatrics, 117* (6), e1163–1169.

15. Philipp, B.L., Merewood, A. & O'Brien, S. (2003). Methadone and breastfeeding: New horizons. *Pediatrics, 111* (6 Pt. 1), 1429–1430.

16. Begg, E.J., Malpas, T.J., Hackett, L.P. & Ilett, K.F. (2001). Distribution of R- and S-methadone into human milk during multiple, medium to high oral dosing. *British Journal of Clinical Pharmacology, 52* (6), 681–685.

17. American Academy of Pediatrics, Committee on Drugs. (1994). The transfer of drugs and other chemicals into human milk. *Pediatrics, 93* (1), 137–150.

18. McCarthy, J.J. & Posey, B.S. (2000). Methadone levels in human milk. *Journal of Human Lactation, 16* (2), 115–120.

19. Jansson, L.M., Choo, R.E., Harrow, C., Velez, M., Schroeder, J.R., Lowe, R. et al. (2007). Concentrations of methadone in breast milk and plasma in the immediate perinatal period. *Journal of Human Lactation, 23* (2), 184–190.

20. Jansson, L.M., Velez, M. & Harrow, C. (2004). Methadone maintenance and lactation: A review of the literature and current management guidelines. *Journal of Human Lactation, 20* (1), 62–71.

21. Geraghty, B., Graham, E.A., Logan, B. & Weiss, E.L. (1997). Methadone levels in breast milk. *Journal of Human Lactation, 13* (3), 227–230.

22. American Academy of Pediatrics, Committee on Drugs. (2001). The transfer of drugs and other chemicals into human milk. *Pediatrics, 108* (3), 776–789.

23. Koren, G., Cairns, J., Chitayat, D., Gaedigk, A. & Leeder, S.J. (2006). Pharmacogenetics of morphine poisoning in a breastfed neonate of a codeine-prescribed mother. *Lancet, 368* (9536), 704.

24. Kahan, M. & Wilson, L. (2002). *Managing Alcohol, Tobacco and Other Drug Problems: A Pocket Guide for Physicians and Nurses.* Toronto: Centre for Addiction and Mental Health.

Tobacco

Cigarette smoke contains over 4,000 chemicals, including cyanide, aluminum, DDT, dieldrin, ammonia, arsenic, formaldehyde, benzene, hydrogen, lead, carbon monoxide, carbon dioxide, tar, chloroform and vinyl chloride.

Despite a decrease in overall smoking rates in Canada, Health Canada estimates that approximately 25 per cent of all pregnant women smoke during their pregnancies.[1] Nicotine is the addictive drug found in cigarettes and has a half-life of two hours.[2] Nicotine crosses the placenta easily and, unlike most drugs (which maintain similar maternal and fetal concentrations), fetal concentrations of nicotine are generally 15 per cent higher than maternal levels.[3]

SUMMARY AND RECOMMENDATIONS

- Cigarette smoking is highly addictive. Despite knowing smoking is harmful during pregnancy and breastfeeding, and despite making an effort, some women are unable to quit. These women should be encouraged to undergo smoking cessation therapy (e.g., nicotine patch, nicotine gum, counselling). If such therapy is unsuccessful, a harm reduction approach is suggested. The mother should be encouraged to reduce the number of cigarettes smoked each day as much as possible, as there is a correlation between dose and fetal/neonatal response (i.e., the more cigarettes smoked, the more potential harm to the fetus or baby).

- If the mother can abstain from smoking for four-hour intervals (i.e., approximately two nicotine half-lives), nicotine concentrations would be expected to fall to one-quarter of their initial level. This means less nicotine and other harmful substances will enter the breast milk.

- To avoid second-hand smoke entering the child's system, no one should ever smoke near the baby.

Fetal effects

Smoking has an adverse effect on fetal growth, and is associated with premature birth and low birth weight. A mean decrease in birth weight of 200 grams is usually associated with babies whose mothers smoked while pregnant.[4]

Preterm premature rupture of membranes has been shown to occur more frequently (1.4 per cent) in women who smoked 20 or more cigarettes per day during pregnancy, while the rate dropped to 0.6 per cent in women who smoked one to five cigarettes per day and to 0.3 per cent in non-smokers.[5]

In addition, a meta-analysis of 13 observational studies (seven case-control and six cohort studies) found that smoking is associated with a two-fold increase in the risk of placental abruptions.[6]

Major malformations

Smoking has not been associated with an increased risk of major malformations.

Spontaneous abortion

Prenatal exposure to tobacco is associated with an increased risk of spontaneous abortion.[4]

Neonatal effects

Studies have reported on the neurotoxic effects of prenatal tobacco exposure, passive addiction and neonatal nicotine withdrawal syndrome (NNWS) in newborns exposed in utero to maternal smoking. NNWS is characterized by irritability, tremors and sleep disturbances, most typically observed in newborns of mothers who smoke heavily.[7]

Also, in a large prospective follow-up study of 24,986 participants, the risk of sudden infant death syndrome (SIDS) was three times higher in children born to mothers who smoked. In addition, the risk of SIDS increased with the number of cigarettes a woman smoked each day during pregnancy, with the greatest risk associated with 10 or more cigarettes smoked daily.[8]

Second-hand smoke must also be taken into account as a health risk to the newborn.

Long-term effects on the child

A study of 5,636 adult men found that, compared to the sons of women who did not smoke while pregnant, those whose mothers did smoke while pregnant had more than a two-fold greater risk of committing a violent crime, or repeatedly committing crimes, even when other biopsychosocial risk factors were controlled.[9]

Breastfeeding

Women who breastfeed and smoke have lower basal prolactin levels, which may lead to a decrease in their milk supply. One study suggests that cigarette smoking significantly reduces breast milk production at two weeks postpartum (i.e., from 514 millilitres per day in mothers who do not smoke to 406 millilitres per day in mothers who do smoke).[10] However, another more recent study detected no change in milk production of mothers who smoked and breastfed their babies.[11]

Although the effects of nicotine are dose dependent, the potential long-term effects on infants exposed to nicotine via breast milk are unknown.

Nicotine is only one component of cigarette smoke; the potential adverse effects on the infant from exposure to the thousands of other chemicals present in cigarette smoke and their passage into breast milk are unknown.

Withdrawal effects on the mother

About 20 percent of people who have established a smoking habit (i.e., smoking on a daily basis for one month) develop nicotine dependence.[12,13] Symptoms of nicotine withdrawal include irritability, restlessness, anxiety, insomnia and fatigue. While these symptoms vanish within a couple of weeks, some people may be unable to concentrate, and have strong cravings to smoke, for weeks or months after quitting smoking.

References

1. Health Canada. (2005). *Healthy Living: Smoking and Your Body—Pregnancy.* Available: www.hc-sc.gc.ca/hl-vs/tobac-tabac/body-corps/preg-gros/index_e.html. Accessed July 10, 2007.

2. Society for Clinical Preventative Health Care. (n.d.). *Clinical Tobacco Intervention Recognition Program.* Vancouver: Author. Available: www.clinicalprevention.ca/ctirp/pharmacy/readings/12stopsmokingmedications.html. Accessed July 13, 2007.

3. Lambers, D.S. & Clark, K.E. (1996). The maternal and fetal physiologic effects of nicotine. *Seminars in Perinatology, 20* (2), 115–126.

4. Pollack, H., Lantz, P.M. & Frohna, J.G. (2000). Maternal smoking and adverse birth outcomes among singletons and twins. *American Journal of Public Health, 90* (3), 395–400.

5. Castles, A., Adams, E.K., Melvin, C.L., Kelsch, C. & Boulton, M.L. (1999). Effects of smoking during pregnancy: Five meta-analyses. *American Journal of Preventive Medicine, 16* (3), 208–215.

6. Ananth, C.V., Smulian, J.C. & Vintzileos, A.M. (1999). Incidence of placental abruption in relation to cigarette smoking and hypertensive disorders during pregnancy: A meta-analysis of observational studies. *Obstetrics and Gynecology, 93* (4), 622–628.

7. Pichini, S. & Garcia-Algar, O. (2006). In utero exposure to smoking and newborn neurobehavior: How to assess neonatal withdrawal syndrome? *Therapeutic Drug Monitoring, 28* (3), 288–290.

8. Wisborg, K., Kesmodel, U., Henriksen, T.B., Olsen, S.F. & Secher, N.J. (2000). A prospective study of smoking during pregnancy and SIDS. *Archives of Disease in Childhood, 83* (3), 203–206.

9. Räsänen, P., Hakko, H., Isohanni, M., Hodgins, S., Järvelin, M. & Tiihonen, J. (1999). Maternal smoking during pregnancy and risk of criminal behavior among adult male offspring in the Northern Finland 1966 Birth Cohort. *American Journal of Psychiatry, 156* (6), 857–862.

10. Ilett, K.F., Hale, T.W., Page-Sharp, M., Kristensen, J.H., Kohan, R. & Hackett, L.P. (2003). Use of nicotine patches in breast-feeding mothers: Transfer of nicotine and cotinine into human milk. *Clinical Pharmacology and Therapeutics, 74* (6), 516–524.

11. Hopkinson, J.M., Schanler, R.J., Fraley, J.K. & Garza, C. (1992). Milk production by mothers of premature infants: Influence of cigarette smoking. *Pediatrics, 90* (6), 934–938.

12. Breslau, N., Johnson, E.O., Hiripi, E. & Kessler, R. (2001). Nicotine dependence in the United States: Prevalence, trends, and smoking persistence. *Archives of General Psychiatry, 58* (9), 810–816.

13. Kessler, D.A, Natanblut, S.L., Wilkenfeld, J.P., Lorraine, C.C., Mayl, S.L., Bernstein, I.B. et al. (1997). Nicotine addiction: A pediatric disease. *Journal of Pediatrics, 130* (4), 518–524.

Resources

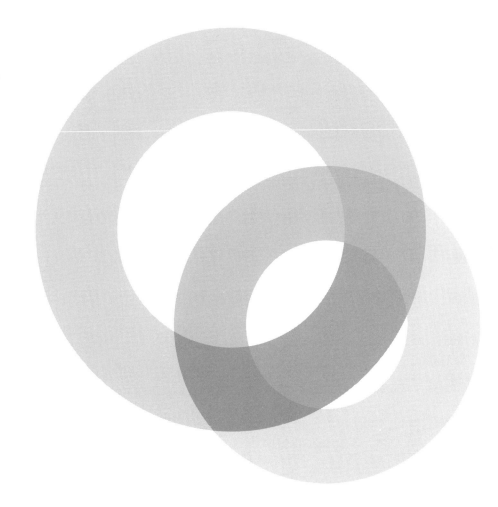

Resources

Motherisk

A clinical, research and teaching program dedicated to antenatal drug, chemical and disease risk counselling. Provides evidence-based teratogen information for health care professionals and updates on Motherisk's continuing reproductive risk research. Offers pregnant, planning and breastfeeding women answers to questions about morning sickness and the risk or safety of medications, herbs, diseases, chemical exposures, radiation and environmental agents.

Website: www.motherisk.org

Alcohol and Substance Use Helpline

Offers information, counselling and referrals about the effects of alcohol and other substances to pregnant and breastfeeding women as well as their families and health care providers.

Tel.: 1 877 FAS-INFO (1 877 327-4636)

Website: www.motherisk.org/women/alcohol.jsp#one

Centre for Addiction and Mental Health (CAMH)

The largest addiction and mental health organization in North America, combining clinical care services, health promotion, education and research. Produces resources—including online and classroom courses, workshops, seminars and publications—for front-line workers in the fields of addiction and mental health, for primary care providers, for helping professionals and for the general public.

Website: www.camh.net

Addiction Clinical Consultation Services (ACCS)

A program serving health and social service professionals including physicians, nurses, psychologists, occupational health staff, social workers, correctional staff, addiction workers and others who work with clients who have alcohol or other substance use problems. Provides advice on the medical complications of alcohol and other drug use; management of clients with addiction problems; counselling for individuals, couples and families; alcohol and other drugs including tobacco, illegal drugs, and prescription and over-the-counter medications; drug interactions; and concurrent disorders.

Tel.: 1 888 720-ACCS (1 888 720-2227)

R. Samuel McLaughlin Addiction and Mental Health Information Centre

Supports Ontarians who find it difficult to access the mental health and addiction systems, in particular, those from diverse communities. Offers a toll-free information line and a telephone support line. Print material, recorded messages and web resources on mental health and substance use problems are available in 16 languages.

Tel.: 1 800 463-6273

E-mail: mclaughlininformation@camh.net

PRIMA (Pregnancy-Related Issues in the Management of Addictions)

Helps health professionals provide obstetric care for pregnant women and new mothers who use substances of abuse, and offers neonatal and pediatric care for children who were exposed to substances in utero. Provides information on the general care of women, including the initial clinical encounter, management of a medical emergency, approaches to care, follow-up visits, infectious diseases and drug toxicology testing.

Website: http://dfcm.utoronto.ca/research/prima/Home.html

Best Start

A maternal, newborn and early child development resource centre that supports service providers across Ontario working on health promotion initiatives to enhance the health of expectant and new parents, newborns and young children. Offers regional workshops and other training opportunities, produces resources to help service providers plan and deliver programs, provides consultations in English and French. Staff answer questions and connect providers with others working on similar initiatives.

Website: www.beststart.org

Canadian Centre on Substance Abuse (CCSA)

Provides evidence-based information and advice aimed at reducing the health, social and economic harms associated with alcohol and other drug use. Dedicated to disseminating information, providing policy guidance, building partnerships and sharing treatment knowledge and best practices related to substance abuse issues, the CCSA works collaboratively with governments, researchers, enforcement agencies, treatment professionals and the private sector to achieve a balanced and holistic approach to addictions that will lead to a healthier and safer Canadian public.

Website: www.ccsa.ca/ccsa/

Canadian Women's Health Network (CWHN)

Builds links among researchers, clinicians, decision-makers, action networks, women, the public and the health care system, and aims to improve the health and lives of girls and women in Canada and the world by collecting, producing and sharing information, resources and strategies. Guided by a woman-centred, holistic vision of women's health, CWHN respects the diverse realities of women's lives and works to end discrimination based on gender, region, race, age, language, religion, sexual orientation or ability, as well as to change inequitable health policies and practices. CWHN functions in English and French, and provides access to health information, resources and research in other languages and alternative formats when possible.

Website: www.cwhn.ca

Healthy Babies

A Health Canada website providing information and tools to help health professionals and other care providers who deliver programs and services to parents and their children. Also provides information to parents on specific topics to reduce the risk of injury and illness and to promote the healthy development of their infants (e.g., how to make environments safer for children, how to reduce the risk of sudden infant death syndrome, why breastfeeding is best for babies and what helps to make breastfeeding a successful experience, how to protect infants from vaccine-preventable diseases).

Website: www.hc-sc.gc.ca/hl-vs/babies-bebes/index_e.html

Pregnets

Aims to decrease the negative consequences of smoking and environmental tobacco smoke on the woman, fetus and child by encouraging health care providers to include brief cessation interventions in routine assessments and health care, and to refer clients who are pregnant or postpartum to existing smoking cessation resources in their community. Using a woman-centred model of care, Pregnets works to eliminate smoking in pregnant and postpartum women by increasing the capacity to quit and remain abstinent. Pregnets provides information on smoking cessation practices for pregnant and postpartum women, a toolkit for health care professionals, a printer-friendly Nicotine Dependency Test and an anonymous online discussion board.

Website: www.pregnets.org

Women for Sobriety (WFS)

Provides support for women trying to overcome alcoholism and other addictions. WFS developed the New Life Program, which encourages building on emotional and spiritual growth to develop a new lifestyle. The program can be used in women's self-help groups as well as in hospitals, clinics, treatment facilities, women centres and wherever people with addiction problems are treated. WFS sets up self-help groups throughout the world, and produces and distributes resources written specifically for women.

Website: www.womenforsobriety.org

Index of Drugs

Index of drugs

Index of drugs

DRUG	SECTION OF BOOK	PAGES
carbamazepine (Tegretol)	Antiepileptics	54–57
Carbolith	Lithium	2, 85–88
cat tranquilizers	Club drugs	75–77
Celexa (citalopram)	Antidepressants	49–53
chalk	Amphetamines	45–48
chlordiazepoxide (Librium)	Benzodiazepines	65–67
chlorpromazine (Largactil)	Antipsychotics	58–61
chronic	Cannabis	71–74, 78
cigarettes	Tobacco	3, 19, 71, 78–79, 95–98
citalopram (Celexa)	Antidepressants	49–53
cleaning fluids	Inhalants	83–84
clomipramine (Anafranil)	Antidepressants	49–53
clonazepam (Rivotril)	Benzodiazepines	65–67
clozapine (Clozaril)	Antipsychotics	58–61
Clozaril (clozapine)	Antipsychotics	58–61
club drugs	Club drugs	75–77
cocaine	Cocaine	3, 78–82
codeine	Opioids	89–94
coffee	Caffeine	68–70
coke	Cocaine	3, 78–82
crack	Cocaine	3, 78–82
crank	Amphetamines	45–48
crystal (crystal methamphetamine)	Amphetamines	45–48
crystal meth	Amphetamines	45–48
D Dalmane (flurazepam)	Benzodiazepines	65–67
delta-9-tetrahydrocannabinol (Marinol)	Cannabis	71–74
delta-9-tetrahydrocannabinol / cannabidiol (Sativex)	Cannabis	71–74
Demerol (meperidine)	Opioids	89–94
Desyrel (trazodone)	Antidepressants	49–53
Dexedrine (dextroamphetamine)	Amphetamines	45–48

Exposure to Psychotropic Medications and Other Substances during Pregnancy and Lactation

Index of drugs

DRUG	SECTION OF BOOK	PAGES
glass	Amphetamines	45–48
grass	Cannabis	71–74, 78
glue	Inhalants	83–84
grievous bodily harm (GHB/gamma-hydroxybutyrate)	Club drugs	75–77
H H (heroin)	Opioids	89–94
Halcion (triazolam)	Benzodiazepines	65–67
Haldol (haloperidol)	Antipsychotics	58–61
haloperidol (Haldol)	Antipsychotics	58–61
hash (hashish)	Cannabis	71–74
hashish	Cannabis	71–74
hash oil	Cannabis	71–74
herb	Cannabis	71–74, 78
heroin	Opioids	89–94
homegrown	Cannabis	71–74, 78
honey oil (hash oil)	Cannabis	71–74
horse (heroin)	Opioids	89–94
hydro	Cannabis	71–74, 78
hydrocodone (Tussionex)	Opioids	89–94
hydromorphone (Dilaudid)	Opioids	89–94
hypnotics	Anxiolytics/sedatives (non-benzodiazepines), Benzodiazepines	1–2, 62–64, 65–67, 76, 91
I ice	Amphetamines	45–48
imipramine (Tofranil)	Antidepressants	49–53
Imovane (zopiclone)	Anxiolytics/sedatives (non-benzodiazepines)	62–64
inhalants	Inhalants	83–84
J jay	Cannabis	71–74, 78
jib	Amphetamines	45–48
joint	Cannabis	71–74, 78

Index of drugs

DRUG	SECTION OF BOOK	PAGES
meth (methadone)	Opioids	7, 89–94
meth (methamphetamine)	Amphetamines	45–48
methadone	Opioids	7, 89–94
methamphetamine	Amphetamines	45–48
methylphenidate (Ritalin)	Amphetamines	45–48
midazolam (Versed)	Benzodiazepines	65–67
mirtazapine (Remeron)	Antidepressants	49–53
Miss Emma (morphine)	Opioids	89–94
MJ	Cannabis	71–74, 78
Mogadon (nitrazepam)	Benzodiazepines	65–67
morph (morphine)	Opioids	89–94
morphine (MS Contin, Statex)	Opioids	89–94
MS Contin (morphine)	Opioids	89–94
N Neurontin (gabapentin)	Antiepileptics	54–57
nicotine	Tobacco	3, 19, 71, 78–79, 95–98
nitrazepam (Mogadon)	Benzodiazepines	65–67
nitrites	Inhalants	83–84
nitrous oxide	Inhalants	83–84
O OC (oxycodone/OxyContin)	Opioids	89–94
olanzapine (Zyprexa)	Antipsychotics	58–61
opioids	Opioids	3, 7, 8, 89–94
oxazepam (Serax)	Benzodiazepines	65–67
oxcarbazepine (Trileptal)	Antiepileptics	54–57
oxy (oxycodone/OxyContin)	Opioids	89–94
oxycodone (Percocet, Percodan, OxyContin)	Opioids	89–94
OxyContin (oxycodone)	Opioids	89–94
P paroxetine (Paxil)	Antidepressants	49–53
party drugs	Club Drugs	75–77

Exposure to Psychotropic Medications and Other Substances during Pregnancy and Lactation

DRUG	SECTION OF BOOK	PAGES
Paxil (paroxetine)	Antidepressants	49–53
penfluridol	Antipsychotics	58–61
pep pills	Amphetamines	45–48
Percocet (oxycodone)	Opioids	89–94
Percodan (oxycodone)	Opioids	89–94
percs (oxycodone)	Opioids	89–94
perphenazine (Trilafon)	Antipsychotics	58–61
phenytoin (Dilantin)	Antiepileptics	54–57
poppers (nitrites)	Inhalants	83–84
pot	Cannabis	71–74, 78
powder lines	Cocaine	3, 78–82
Prozac (fluoxetine)	Antidepressants	49–53
Q quetiapine (Seroquel)	Antipsychotics	58–61
R reefer	Cannabis	71–74, 78
Remeron (mirtazapine)	Antidepressants	49–53
Restoril (temazepam)	Benzodiazepines	65–67
Risperdal (risperidone)	Antipsychotics	58–61
risperidone (Risperdal)	Antipsychotics	58–61
Ritalin (methylphenidate)	Amphetamines	45–48
Rivotril (clonazepam)	Benzodiazepines	65–67
roachies (flunitrazepam/Rohypnol)	Club drugs, Benzodiazepines	65–67, 75–77
rock (crack cocaine)	Cocaine	3, 78–82
Rohypnol (flunitrazepam)	Club drugs, Benzodiazepines	65–67, 75–77
roofies (flunitrazepam/Rohypnol)	Club drugs, Benzodiazepines	65–67, 75–77
room odourizers	Inhalants	83–84
rope, rophies, ruffies (flunitrazepam/Rohypnol)	Club drugs, Benzodiazepines	65–67, 75–77
Rush (nitrites)	Inhalants	83–84

Index of drugs

DRUG	SECTION OF BOOK	PAGES
tranks	Benzodiazepines	1–2, 62, 65–67, 76, 91
trazodone (Desyrel)	Antidepressants	49–53
triazolam (Halcion)	Benzodiazepines	65–67
tricyclics	Antidepressants	49–53
Trilafon (perphenazine)	Antipsychotics	58–61
Trileptal (oxcarbazepine)	Antiepileptics	54–57
Tussionex (hydrocodone)	Opioids	89–94
Tylenol 3 (codeine)	Opioids	89–94
typical antipsychotics	Antipsychotics	54–57
U uppers	Amphetamines	45–48
V Valium (diazepam)	Benzodiazepines	65–67
valproate (Epival)	Antiepileptics	54–57
valproic acid (Epival)	Antiepileptics	54–57
VCR head cleaner	Inhalants	83–84
venlafaxine (Effexor)	Antidepressants	49–53
Versed (midazolam)	Benzodiazepines	65–67
vitamin K (ketamine)	Club drugs	75–77
W weed	Cannabis	71–74, 78
weed oil (hash oil)	Cannabis	71–74
Wellbutrin (bupropion)	Antidepressants	49–53
whippets (nitrous oxide)	Inhalants	83–84
X Xanax (alprazolam)	Benzodiazepines	65–67
XTC (MDMA/ecstacy)	Club drugs	75–77
Z Zoloft (sertraline)	Antidepressants	49–53
zopiclone (Imovane)	Anxiolytics/sedatives (non-benzodiazepines)	62–64
Zyban (bupropion)	Antidepressants	49–53
Zyprexa (olanzapine)	Antipsychotics	58–61